Nursing Dosage Calculation Workbook

24 Categories of Problems from Basic to Advanced

Authors:

Bradley J. Wojcik, PharmD

Chase Hassen

Disclaimer:

Although the author and publisher have made every effort to ensure that the information in this book was correct at press time, the author and publisher do not assume and hereby disclaim any liability to any party for any loss, damage, or disruption caused by errors or omissions, whether such errors or omissions result from negligence, accident, or any other cause.

This book is not intended as a substitute for the medical advice of physicians. The reader should regularly consult a physician in matters relating to his/her health and particularly with respect to any symptoms that may require diagnosis or medical attention.

All rights reserved. No part of this publication may be reproduced, distributed, or transmitted in any form or by any means, including photocopying, recording, or other electronic or mechanical methods, without the prior written permission of the publisher, except in the case of brief quotations embodied in critical reviews and certain other noncommercial uses permitted by copyright law.

NCLEX®, NCLEX®-RN, and NCLEX®-PN are registered trademarks of the National Council of State Boards of Nursing, Inc. They hold no affiliation with this product.

Some images within this book are either royalty-free images, used under license from their respective copyright holders, or images that are in the public domain.

© **Copyright 2019 by Chase Hassen & Bradley J. Wojcik, PharmD. All rights reserved.** | **ISBN:** 9781797987415

Join the FB Group to get Free Video Lessons, Homework and Quizzes!

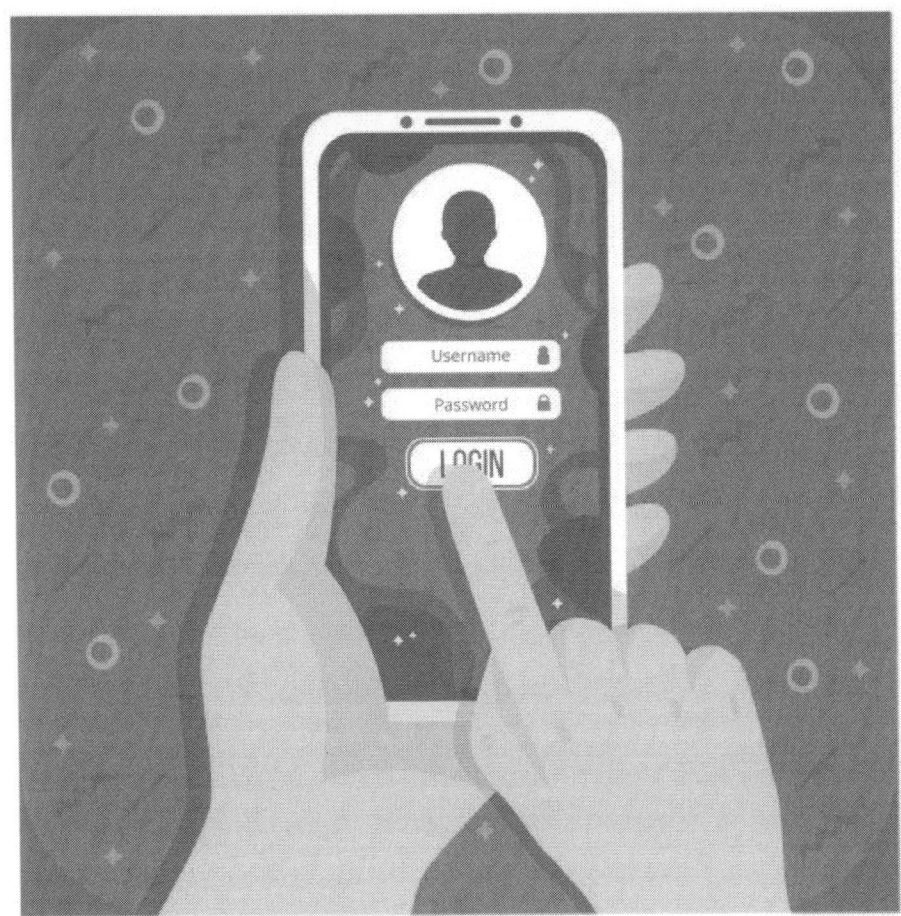

Visit: www.nursesuperhero.com/dw to join now!

Table of Contents

Introduction 7

Unit 1: Basic Math and Military Time 10
- Chapter 1 Rounding Numbers 11
- Chapter 2 Roman Numerals 12
- Chapter 3 Scientific Notation 13
- Chapter 4 Military Time 15

Unit 2: Unit Conversions 17
- Chapter 5 Unit Conversions Within the Metric System 18
- Chapter 6 Unit Conversions Within the Household System 19
- Chapter 7 Unit Conversions Between Metric, Household and Apothecary Systems 20

Unit 3: Dosage Calculations 21
- Chapter 8 Dosage Calculations Level 1 22
- Chapter 9 Dosage Calculations Level 2 24
- Chapter 10 Dosage Calculations Level 3 29
- Chapter 11 Body Surface Area Dosing Calculations 36
- Chapter 12 Pediatric Dosing Problems 40
- Chapter 13 Pediatric Maintenance Fluid Replacement Calculations 43

Unit 4: IV Flow Rate Calculations 45
- Chapter 14 IV Flow Rate Calculations Level I 46
- Chapter 15 IV Flow Rate Calculations Level 2 50
- Chapter 16 IV Flow Rate Adjustments 57
- Chapter 17 Heparin Infusion and Adjustment Calculations 62

Unit 5: Percent and Ratio Strength Calculations 69
- Chapter 18 Percent 70
- Chapter 19 Percent Strength 71
- Chapter 20 Percent Change 73
- Chapter 21 Ratio Strength 76

Unit 6: Miscellaneous Subjects 77
- Chapter 22 Reconstitution Calculations 78

Chapter 23 Conversions Between mg and mEq 81

Chapter 24 Dosage Calculations Puzzles 82

Chapter 25 Self-Assessment Exam 84

A Final Note 92

List of Abbreviations and Symbols 93

Answers to Exercises 94

Chapter 1 Rounding Numbers 94

Chapter 2 Roman Numerals 95

Chapter 3 Scientific Notation 96

Chapter 4 Military Time 98

Chapter 5 Unit Conversions Within the Metric System 100

Chapter 6 Unit Conversions Within the Household System 101

Chapter 7 Unit Conversions Between Metric, Household and Apothecary Systems 102

Chapter 8 Dosage Calculations Level 1 103

Chapter 9 Dosage Calculations Level 2 105

Chapter 10 Dosage Calculations Level 3 109

Chapter 11 BSA Calculation Problems 115

Chapter 12 Pediatric Dosing Problems 118

Chapter 13 Pediatric Maintenance Fluid Replacement Calculations 122

Chapter 14 IV Flow Rate Calculations Level I 124

Chapter 15 IV Flow Rate Calculations Level 2 128

Chapter 16 IV Flow Rate Adjustments 133

Chapter 17 Heparin Infusion and Adjustment Calculations 137

Chapter 18 Percent 145

Chapter 19 Percent Strength 146

Chapter 20 Percent Change 148

Chapter 21 Ratio Strength 150

Chapter 22 Reconstitution Calculations 151

Chapter 23 Conversions Between mg and mEq 153

Chapter 24 Dosage Calculations Puzzles 154

Chapter 25 Self-Assessment Exam 156

Introduction

Welcome to our dosage calculation workbook with over 777 problems for your enjoyment! This book is intended to be used as an advanced workbook supplement to Wojcik, B & Hassen, C (2018) *Dosage calculations for nursing students: Master dosage calculations in 24 hours the safe & easy way without formulas!* ISBN 9781725638839 (DCFNS). In addition to covering all the problems in DCFNS, this book contains advanced dosage and IV flow rate problems along with the following new categories:

- Body Surface Area Dosing Calculations
- Pediatric Dosing Calculations
- Pediatric Maintenance Fluid Replacement Calculations
- IV Flow Rate Adjustment Calculations
- Heparin Infusion and Adjustment Calculations
- Reconstitution Calculations

To get the most out of this book:

- Read and understand the concepts presented in DCFNS.
- Do the problems in DCFNS.
- Identify the areas where you are having problems and do the practice problems in this book.
- Work on the advanced dosage and IV flow rate problems as well as the new categories.

This book is organized into the following six units:

Unit 1: Basic Math Problems and Military Time

- Rounding Numbers
- Roman Numerals
- Scientific Notation
- Military Time

These subjects are covered in DCFNS and should serve as review questions.

Unit 2: Conversions

- Unit Conversions Within the Metric System
- Unit Conversions Within the Household System
- Unit Conversions Between the Metric, Household and Apothecary Systems

These subjects are covered in DCFNS.

Unit 3: Dosage Calculations

- Dosage Calculations Level 1
- Dosage Calculations Level 2
- Dosage Calculations Level 3
- Body Surface Area Dosing Calculations
- Pediatric Dosing Calculations
- Pediatric Maintenance Fluid Replacement Calculations

DCFNS was designed to provide a sound foundation on setting up and solving basic dosage calculations. This unit builds on that foundation by providing basic problems along with advanced dosage problems, which are in the Level 3 section. This unit also covers the specific subjects of Body Surface Area Calculations, Pediatric Dosing Calculations and Pediatric Maintenance Fluid Replacement Calculations.

Unit 4: IV Flow Rate Calculations

- IV Flow Rate Calculations Level 1
- IV Flow Rate Calculations Level 2
- IV Flow Rate Adjustment Calculations
- Heparin Infusion and Adjustment Calculations

DCFNS was designed to provide a basic knowledge of how to set up and solve IV flow rate problems. This unit builds on that foundation by first providing a review of the basic problems in Level 1, then more advanced problems in Level 2. This unit also covers the new subjects of IV Flow Rate Adjustment Calculations and Heparin Infusion and Adjustment Calculations.

Unit 5: Percent and Ratio Strength Calculations

- Percent
- Percent Strength
- Percent Change
- Ratio Strength

This unit reinforces the material in DCFNS.

Unit 6: Miscellaneous Subjects

- Reconstitution Calculations
- Conversions Between mg and mEq
- Dosage Calculation Puzzles
- Self-Assessment Exam
- List of Abbreviations and Symbols

This unit has the new subjects of Reconstitution Calculations and Dosage Calculations Puzzles. The self-assessment exam in this book is longer and more involved than DCFNS and is designed to give an accurate assessment of your skills. A list of abbreviations and symbols is included at the end.

Rounding rules for this book, unless otherwise stated:

- In general, round calculations at the end.
- All drops/minute calculations are to be rounded to the nearest full drop.
- All mL/h calculations are to be rounded to the nearest tenth mL/h unless otherwise stated.
- mL doses less than 1 mL are rounded to the nearest hundredth mL.
- mL doses greater than or equal to 1 mL are rounded to the nearest tenth mL.
- When rounding the final answer to the nearest tenth or hundredth, if the final digit after the decimal point is zero, omit it. For example: 5.03 mL rounded to the nearest tenth is 5.0 mL but drop the zero and write as 5 mL.

Enjoy the book!

-Brad Wojcik & Chase Hassen

Unit 1: Basic Math and Military Time

Chapter 1: Rounding
Corresponding Chapter and pages in DCFNS: Chapter 4, pp. 16-17.
Importance: 10/10. If you don't understand rounding, you will not pass your dosage calculations class.

Chapter 2: Roman Numerals
Corresponding Chapter and pages in DCFNS: Chapter 5, pp. 18-22.
Importance: 5/10. You should know the basics and at least 1-20. It is also good to know for everyday life.

Chapter 3: Scientific Notation
Corresponding Chapter and pages in DCFNS: Chapter 6, pp. 23-25.
Importance: 3/10. It is unlikely you will need this for dosage calculations, but you will need to know this if you take any chemistry classes. It is easy to learn, so you should learn it.

Chapter 4: Military Time
Corresponding Chapter and pages in DCFNS: Chapter 7, pp. 26-27.
Importance: 10/10. You must know this.

Chapter 1
Rounding Numbers
(Include trailing zeros in this exercise.)

Problem	Round to the Nearest Tenth	Rounded Number		Round to the Nearest Hundredth	Rounded Number
1	6.47	6.5	26	89.568	89.568
2	3.15	3.2	27	45.789	45.889
3	0.06	0.1	28	1.005	1.005
4	23.49	23.49	29	2.895	2.895
5	6.999	6.999	30	3.997	3.997
6	1.447	1.447	31	7.894	7.894
7	16.24	16.24	32	3.433	3.433
8	149.10	149.10	33	2.222	2.222
9	10.011	10.011	34	1.111	1.111
10	9.97	9.97	35	8.895	8.895
11	1001.89	1001.89	36	29.999	29.999
12	21.46	21.46	37	56.451	56.451
13	0.059	0.059	38	3.4723	3.4723
14	0.0010	0.0010	39	6.7754	6.7754
15	6.239	6.239	40	0.099	0.099
16	4.4499	4.4499	41	5.773	5.773
17	5.97	5.97	42	9.065	9.065
18	6.37	6.4	43	7.436	7.436
19	78.467	78.467	44	61.7712	61.7712
20	4.449	4.449	45	73.612	73.612
21	97.89	97.89	46	9.713	9.713
22	1.01	1.01	47	4.59	4.6
23	5.67	5.7	48	66.7812	66.7812
24	23.2323	23.2323	49	0.795	0.995
25	64.0	64.0	50	3.912	3.912

Chapter 2
Roman Numerals

Fill in the blanks with the corresponding Roman numeral.

Problem	Number	Roman Numeral	Prob #	Number	Roman Numeral
1	6	VI	11	8	VIII
2	9	IX	12	200	CC
3	50	L	13	178	CLXVIII
4	2	II	14	99	IC
5	49	IL	15	30	XXX
6	9	IX	16	35	XXXV
7	22	XXII	17	½	S
8	100	C	18	4	IV
9	20	XX	19	2004	MMIV
10	33	XXXIII	20	36	XXXVI

Fill in the blanks with the corresponding number.

Problem	Roman Numeral	Number	Prob #	Roman Numeral	Number
21	V	5	31	XLIV	
22	IV	4	32	DL	
23	XX	20	33	CDL	
24	XC	90	34	III	
25	CXI	111	35	VIII	
26	XXXIV	34	36	LXVI	
27	MCM	1	37	CC	
28	SS		38	CXC	
29	XLI		39	MMXIX	
30	CI		40	XL	

Chapter 3
Scientific Notation

Convert the following numbers to scientific notation.

Problem	Number	Coefficient	# of Places from New Decimal Point to end of Original Number	Coefficient X 10 Raised to the Number of Places the Decimal Point was Moved
Example	47,000	4.7	4	4.7×10^4
1	64,500	6.45	4	6.45×10^4
2	23,000,000	2.3	7	2.3×10^7
3	14,000	1.4	4	1.4×10^4
4	237,400,000	2.374	8	2.374×10^8
5	1,000,100	1.0001	6	1.0001×10^6
6	175,000	1.75	5	1.75×10^5
7	63,500,000	6.35	7	6.35×10^7
8	6,023,000,000	6.023	9	6.023×10^9
9	700,000	7.0	5	7.0×10^5
10	45,020,000	4.502	7	4.502×10^7

Convert the following decimal numbers to scientific notation.

Problem	Decimal Number	Coefficient	# of Places from New Decimal Point to Original Decimal Point	Coefficient X 10 Raised to the Negative Number of Places the Decimal Point was Moved
Example	0.031	3.1	2	3.1×10^{-2}
11	0.000167	1.67	4	1.67×10^{-4}
12	0.000061	6.1	5	6.1×10^{-5}
13	0.0004068	4.068	4	4.068×10^{-4}
14	0.0001975	1.975	4	1.975×10^{-4}
15	0.0002001	2.001	4	2.001×10^{-4}
16	0.000045	4.5	5	4.5×10^{-5}
17	0.00000052	5.2	7	5.2×10^{-7}
18	0.000068	6.8	5	6.8×10^{-5}
19	0.001983	1.983	3	1.983×10^{-3}
20	0.0024	2.4	3	2.4×10^{-3}

Convert the following numbers from scientific notation to numbers.

Problem	Scientific Notation	Coefficient	Exponent	# of Places to Move the Decimal Point to the Right	Number
Example	1.42×10^7	1.42	7	7	14,200,000
21	3.8×10^4	3.8	4	4	38,000
22	4×10^5	4	5	5	400000
23	3.01×10^6	3.01	6	6	3,010,000
24	3.05×10^4	3.05	4	4	30,500
25	2.79×10^8	2.79	8	8	279,000,000
26	8.99×10^5	8.99	5	5	899,000
27	3.78×10^8	3.78	8	8	378,000,000
28	2.0×10^8	2.0	8	8	200,000,000
29	8.56×10^5	8.56	5	5	856,000
30	2.31×10^7	2.31	7	7	23,100,000

Convert the following decimal numbers from scientific notation to decimal numbers.

Problem	Scientific Notation	Coefficient	Exponent	# of Places to Move the Decimal Point to the Left	Decimal Number
Example	3.04×10^{-4}	3.04	-4	4	0.000304
31	9.4×10^{-6}	9.4	-6	6	0.0000094
32	2.81×10^{-5}	2.81	-5	5	0.0000281
33	3.5×10^{-6}	3.5	-6	6	0.0000035
34	6.95×10^{-8}	6.95	-8	8	0.0000000695
35	3.3×10^{-9}	3.3	-9	9	0.0000000033
36	9.00×10^{-4}	9.0	-4	4	0.0009
37	1.42×10^{-3}	1.42	-3	3	0.00142
38	2.02×10^{-3}	2.02	-3	3	0.00202
39	9.6×10^{-7}	9.6	-7	7	0.00000096
40	5.4×10^{-5}	5.4	-5	5	0.000054

Chapter 4
Military Time

Convert the following civilian times to military time.

1) 3:25 AM   0325
2) 11:35 AM   1135
3) 2:29 PM   1429
4) 10:20 PM   2220
5) 4:00 PM   1600

Convert the following military times to civilian times.

6) 0318   3:18 am
7) 2309   11:09 pm
8) 1004   10:04 am
9) 1615   4:15 pm
10) 1309   1:09 pm

11) An IV was started at 1000 and ended at 3:30 PM. How long did it run in hours and minutes?

5:30

12) A patient was admitted at 0900 on Tuesday and was discharged at 2:30 PM on the following day. How many hours did the patient spend in the hospital?

29 1/2

13) A civilian time day has 24 hours. How many hours does a military time day have?

24

14) You start work at 0700 at your hospital in California and take a lunch break at noon. You phone your friend in New York during lunch and after visiting for a while she looks at her watch and says, "It is 1530, I have to get back to work." What time is it in California?

12:30

15) You have the day off and plan to run some errands. You leave the house at 0830, drive for 20 minutes to the coffee shop, spend 30 minutes enjoying your coffee, arrive at the grocery store at 9:45 AM, spend 30 minutes shopping, then arrive home 15 minutes after finishing shopping. What time is it in military time?

1030

16) You have an order for 1 tablet PO q 8 h. You give the first dose at 0800. What time in military time will you give the next two doses?

1500   2300

17) You start an IV at 1000 to run for 4 hours. What time in civilian time will it end?

2:00pm

18) You have an order for 1 capsule PO q 6 h. You administer the first dose at 11:00 AM. What time in military time will you administer the third dose?

5:00pm

19) Your cat is normally fed at 1700, but due to excessive meowing, you feed her at 4:30 PM. How many minutes early was she fed?

30

20) You start an IV at 2300 on Monday and it finishes at 0530 on Tuesday. How long did it run?

6:30

Unit 2: Unit Conversions

Chapter 5: Unit Conversions within the Metric System.
Corresponding Chapter and pages in DCFNS: Chapter 1, pp. 10-11. Chapter 8, pp. 32-35.
Importance: 10/10. If you don't know this, you will flunk nursing school.

Chapter 6: Unit Conversions within the Household System.
Corresponding Chapter and pages in DCFNS: Chapter 2, p. 12 Chapter 8, pp. 32-35.
Importance: 9/10.

Chapter 7: Unit Conversions Between Metric, Household and Apothecary Systems
Corresponding Chapter and pages in DCFNS: Chapter 8, pp. 32-33.
Importance: 10/10.

This unit covers the basics of dimensional analysis and will set you up for success in the remaining chapters.

Chapter 5
Unit Conversions Within the Metric System

Problem	Given to be Converted	Conversion Factor	Units of the Answer	
Example	2.5 g	1000 mg/g =	2500 mg	
1	1.3 g	1000 mg/g =	1300	mg
2	45 mL	1000 mL/L =	0.045	L
3	25 mL	=		dL
4	65 mg	1000 mg/g =	065	g
5	4 cm	=		mm
6	340 mcg	=		mg
7	590 g	=		kg
8	7.8 g	=		mg
9	2.1 L	=		mL
10	98 mm	=		cm
11	6 mcg	=		mg
12	800 mL	=		L
13	5 mL	=		L
14	87 mcg	=		mg
15	650 mcg	=		mg
16	6700 mcg	=		g
17	5 mg	=		mcg
18	78,000 mcg	=		g
19	0.013 L	=		dL
20	2.2 kg	=		g
21	145 mcg	=		mg
22	24 mL	=		L
23	1.01 m	=		cm
24	250 mcg	=		mg
25	3750 g	=		kg
26	45 cm	=		m
27	4.1 L	=		mL
28	100 mL	=		L
29	610 mL	=		dL
30	1.05 L	=		mL

Chapter 6
Unit Conversions Within the Household System

Problem	Given to be Converted	Conversion Factor	Units of the Answer
Example	2 cups	8 fl oz/cup =	16 fl oz
1	2 fl oz	=	tbs
2	0.5 pt	=	fl oz
3	2 gal	=	qt
4	8 oz	=	lb
5	12 fl oz	=	cup
6	2 fl oz	=	tsp
7	6 tsp	=	tbs
8	1 cup	=	fl oz
9	4 fl oz	=	cup
10	1 cup	=	pt
11	2 pt	=	gal
12	1 gal	=	pt
13	4 tsp	=	fl oz
14	4 fl oz	=	tbs
15	2 tsp	=	tbs
16	2 qt	=	cups
17	2 cups	=	fl oz
18	6 tsp	=	fl oz
19	4 pt	=	qt
20	32 oz	=	lb
21	1 pt	=	fl oz
22	3 fl oz	=	tbs
23	6 fl oz	=	tbs
24	2 tbs	=	tsp
25	3 cups	=	pt
26	1 fl oz	=	tsp
27	8 fl oz	=	pt
28	0.5 qt	=	fl oz
29	1 gal	=	fl oz
30	4 cups	=	pt

Chapter 7
Unit Conversions Between Metric, Household and Apothecary Systems

Note: Use 1 gr = 60 mg for these conversions. This differs from DCFNS, which uses 1 gr = 65 mg.

Problem	Given to be Converted	Conversion Factor	Units of the Answer
Example	5 in	2.54 cm/in =	12.7 cm
1	2 gr	=	mg
2	45 lb	=	kg
3	1.5 cup	=	mL
4	60 mL	=	fl oz
5	7 in	=	cm
6	200 g	=	lb
7	3 tsp	=	mL
8	90 mL	=	cup
9	3.5 fl oz	=	mL
10	98 mm	=	in
11	3 gr	=	mg
12	2 tsp	=	mL
13	1.5 fl oz	=	mL
14	4 gr	=	mg
15	18 in	=	cm
16	3 fl oz	=	mL
17	2 tbs	=	mL
18	0.5 pt	=	mL
19	2.2 kg	=	lb
20	120 mg	=	gr
21	90 mL	=	fl oz
22	180 mg	=	gr
23	4 fl oz	=	mL
24	700 g	=	lb
25	180 mL	=	fl oz
26	2 cups	=	fl oz
27	454 g	=	lb
28	5 gr	=	mg

Unit 3: Dosage Calculations

Chapter 8: Dosage Calculations Level 1
Corresponding Chapter and pages in DCFNS: Chapter 9, pp. 36-37.
Importance: 10/10. These are one step basic calculations. You must know this.

Chapter 9: Dosage Calculations Level 2
Corresponding Chapter and pages in DCFNS: Chapter 9, pp. 36-37.
Importance: 10/10. These problems are a bit more involved than the level 1 problems. You must know this material.

Chapter 10: Dosage Calculations Level 3
Corresponding Chapter and pages in DCFNS: Chapter 9, pp. 36-37.
Importance: 10/10. These problems reinforce your ability to utilize the correct information to set up and solve complicated dosage problems. It is important to practice these problems to gain confidence when it comes test time, and later in clinical settings.

Chapter 11: Body Surface Area Dosing Calculations
Corresponding Chapter and pages in DCFNS: None. New material for this book.
Importance: 9/10 for nursing school testing. 5/10 for real life. It is most important to understand what BSA means. You will probably be required to do some of these calculations on nursing school tests, but in the field, you will probably rely on a BSA calculation app. There are several different methods to calculate BSA, but only one method is easily calculated manually.

Chapter 12: Pediatric Dosing Problems
Corresponding Chapter and pages in DCFNS: Chapter 9, pp. 36-37. The actual math is the same in pediatric dosage problems, the difference lies in the types of questions asked. Nursing school pediatric dosing questions seem to focus on dosing ranges, with anything out of range being labeled "unsafe". Follow the instructions on your individual tests, but in real life, do a little research before informing the prescriber that he/she has ordered an unsafe dose.
Importance: 9/10 for nursing school testing. 5-10/10 for real life depending on your area of practice.

Chapter 13: Pediatric Maintenance Fluid Replacement Calculations
Corresponding Chapter and pages in DCFNS: None. New material for this book.
Importance: 9/10 for nursing school testing.

Chapter 8
Dosage Calculations Level 1

Problem	Order	Available	Administer
Example	50 mg	25 mg/mL	50 mg (1 mL/25mg) = 2 mL
1	150 mg	50 mg/mL	
2	500 mg	250 mg capsules	
3	50 mcg	100 mcg/mL	
4	0.5 g	0.25 g tab	
5	10 mg	20 mg/5 mL	
6	0.25 mg	0.125 mg tabs	
7	600 mg	300 mg/2 mL	
8	7.5 mg	5 mg scored tabs	
9	30 mg	15 mg/mL	
10	0.125 mg	0.25 mg/mL	
11	75 mg	50 mg/mL	
12	1 g	0.25 g tab	
13	50 mcg	200 mcg/mL	
14	1000 mg	500 mg tabs	
15	1 mg	10 mg/mL	
16	90 mg	60 mg/mL	
17	250 mg	100 mg/mL	
18	45 mg	50 mg/mL	
19	0.25 g	0.5 g scored tabs	
20	6 mg	3 mg/2 mL	
21	100 mcg	25 mcg/mL	
22	90 mg	200 mg/mL	
23	8.5 mg	2 mg/mL	
24	1 mg	0.5 mg/mL	
25	15 mg	5 mg/5 mL	
26	90 mg	20 mg/mL	
27	0.6 mg	0.3 mg tabs	

Problem	Order	Available	Administer
28	200 mcg	100 mcg/tab	
29	50 mg	100 mg/mL	
30	150 mcg	50 mcg/mL	
31	25 mg	12.5 mg/5 mL	
32	3 mg	6 mg scored tab	
33	20 mg	5 mg/mL	
34	250 mcg	125 mcg tabs	
35	75 mg	150 mg/mL	
36	3 mcg	1 mcg/mL	
37	30 mg	10 mg/5 mL	
38	5 mg	10 mg scored tab	
39	7.5 mg	5 mg/mL	
40	0.3 mg	0.1 mg tab	
41	250 mg	100 mg/mL	
42	3.5 mg	1 mg/mL	
43	480 mg	400 mg/5 mL	
44	30 mg	150 mg/10 mL	
45	500 mg	250 mg capsule	
46	75 mg	25 mg/mL	
47	1000 mg	500 mg/2 mL	
48	20 mEq	10 mEq tab	
49	7.5 mg	5 mg/scored tab	
50	200 mg	100 mg capsule	
51	5 mg	10 mg/mL	
52	500 mg	250 mg/5 mL	
53	20 mEq	20 mEq tab	
54	2 mg	1 mg scored tab	
55	25 mg	50 mg scored tab	
56	250 mg	125 mg/mL	
57	7 mcg	10 mcg/10 mL	
58	200 mg	100 mg capsule	

Chapter 9
Dosage Calculations Level 2

1) The NP has ordered 100 mg IM b.i.d. of a drug which is available in 5 mL vials labeled 50 mg/mL. How many mL will you administer per dose?

2) You have an order for 0.25 mg of levothyroxine which is available in 125 mcg scored tablets. How many tablets will you administer?

3) The physician has ordered drug xyz 50 mg/day IV divided into 2 doses. The pharmacy sends a 5 mL vial which contains drug xyz in a concentration of 100 mg/mL. How many mL will you administer for each dose?

4) Your 45 YO patient who weighs 178 lb has been ordered drug abc 100 mg/day IV divided into 4 doses. Drug abc is available in 10 mL vials containing 50 mg/mL. How many mL will you administer per dose?

5) The MD has ordered 100 mg PO t.i.d. of a drug which is available in 20 mL vials containing 50 mg/mL. How many mL will be administered each day?

6) The provider has ordered 50 mcg/day PO divided into 2 doses. You have available 0.025 mg tablets. How many tablets will you administer per dose?

7) Your 67 YO patient has an order for 200 mg IM q 4 h. The drug is available as 100 mg/mL. How many mL will you administer per dose?

8) The NP has ordered 1 g/day IV divided into 4 doses of a drug which is available in 20 mL vials containing 100 mg/mL. How many mL/dose will you administer?

9) You have an order to administer a 400 mg dose IM of a drug which is available in 10 mL vials containing 1 g. How many mL will you administer?

10) You have an order for 0.125 mg PO of a drug which is available in 125 mcg tablets. How many tablets do you administer?

11) Your patient has been ordered 500 mg IV q 6 h of a drug which is available in 20 mL vials containing 25 mg/mL. How many mL will be administered in 24 hours?

12) The order is for 1 g PO and you have 250 mg capsules available. How many capsules will you administer?

13) You have an order for 500 mcg IV of drug xyz which is available in 5 mL vials labeled 0.25 mg/mL. How many mL will you administer?

14) The physician has ordered 1000 mg/day PO divided into 2 doses of a drug which is available in 250 mg capsules. How many capsules will you administer per dose?

15) Your patient has an order for 1.5 mg IV of a drug which is available in 5 mL vials containing 500 mcg/mL. How many mL will you administer?

16) Your patient is to receive 12.5 mg PO q.i.d. You have 25 mg scored tablets available. How many tablets will the patient receive for each dose?

17) Your patient is to receive 120 mL of a commercial formula via G-Tube q.i.d. The formula is available in 240 mL containers. How many containers will be administered each day?

18) The healthcare provider has ordered 100 mg/day IV divided into 4 doses. You have a 5 mL vial labeled 50 mg/mL. How many mL will you administer per dose?

19) The order is for 0.5 g PO b.i.d. You have 250 mg capsules available. How many capsules will be administered per day?

20) Your patient has an order for 600 mg/day IV divided into 4 doses. You have available a 10 mL vial containing 500 mg of the drug. How many mL will you administer per dose?

21) The order is 500 mcg IV. On hand you have a 2 mL vial containing 1 mg/mL. How many mL will you administer?

22) The PA has ordered 900 mcg IM of a drug which is available in 1 mL vials containing 2 mg/mL. How many mL will you administer?

23) The healthcare provider has ordered 4.5 mg IV t.i.d. for your patient. The drug is available in 10 mL vials containing 10 mg/mL. How many mL will you draw up to administer one dose?

24) The NP has ordered 3 mg IV for your 189 lb patient. The drug is available in 10 mL vials containing 500 mcg/mL. How many mL will you administer?

25) Your patient has an order for 15 mg PO of a drug to be administer at 2100. You have available 7.5 mg capsules. How many capsules will you administer?

26) The physician has ordered 35 mg IV of a drug which is available in 5 mL vials containing 20 mg/mL. How many mL will you administer?

27) The physician has ordered 0.8 mg IV q 2 h for 2 doses. You have available 5 mL vials containing 0.4 mg/mL. How many mL will you administer for one dose?

28) Your pediatric patient will be going home with a 150 mL bottle of amoxicillin 250 mg/5 mL with instructions for 5 mL to be given PO q 8 h. How long will the bottle last?

29) The physician has ordered 100 mg/day IM divided into 2 doses. You have a 1 mL vial labeled 50 mg/mL. How many mL will you administer per dose?

30) You have an order for 1 g/day PO divided into 2 doses. You have 250 mg tablets available. How many tablets will you administer per dose?

Chapter 10
Dosage Calculations Level 3

1) A 74 kg patient is scheduled for a PCI and will receive an IV bolus dose of abciximab 0.25 mg/kg followed immediately by an infusion of the drug. The abciximab is available in 5 mL vials containing 2 mg/mL. How many mL will you administer for the bolus?

2) A 6 YO child weighing 50 lb is diagnosed with bacterial sinusitis and is prescribed azithromycin 10 mg/kg PO once daily for 3 days. Azithromycin oral suspension is available in 15, 22.5 and 30 mL bottles containing 200 mg/5 mL. How many mL will you administer?

3) A 172 lb patient with atrial fibrillation is to receive an initial IV bolus of verapamil 0.075 mg/kg over at least 2 minutes. The drug is available in 4 mL vials containing 2.5 mg/mL. How many mL will you administer?

4) A 60 kg patient is to receive a single IV dose of ondansetron 0.15 mg/kg, in addition to other drugs, for prevention of chemotherapy-induced nausea and vomiting. Ondansetron is available in a MDV of 40 mg/ 20mL. How many mL will you administer?

5) A 6 YO 42 lb child with acute otitis media (AOM) is to receive oral amoxicillin 80 mg/kg/day divided every 12 hours. The amoxicillin is available in 75 mL bottles containing 400 mg/5 mL. How many mL will you administer per dose?

6) A 72 kg male diagnosed with bacterial meningitis has an order for gentamicin 5 mg/kg/day IV in divided doses every 8 hours. How many mg will you administer for each dose?

7) A 12-month-old 22 lb child has been prescribed a maintenance dose of digoxin 10 mcg/kg/day PO administered in equal divided doses twice daily. Digoxin elixir is available in 60 mL bottles containing 50 mcg/mL. How many mL will you administer per dose?

8) A 51 YO 145 lb patient diagnosed with meningitis has an order for amikacin 5 mg/kg IV every 8 hours for 14 days. The amikacin is available in 2 mL vials containing 500 mg. How many mL will you administer each dose?

9) A 174 lb patient is to receive cephalexin 500 mg PO b.i.d. The drug is available in 250 mg capsules. How many capsules will the patient receive in a 24-hour period?

10) A 45 YO 152 lb adult has an order for ceftazidime 90 mg/kg/day IV in divided doses every 8 hours. How many mg will you administer per dose?

11) A 4 YO 38 lb child with hypertension has be ordered furosemide 1 mg/kg/dose PO twice daily. Furosemide oral solution is available in 60 mL bottles containing 10 mg/mL. How many mL will you administer each dose?

12) A 145 lb patient is to receive a single IV dose of ondansetron 0.15 mg/kg, in addition to other drugs, for prevention of chemotherapy-induced nausea and vomiting. Ondansetron is available in a 20 mL MDV of 2 mg/mL. How many mL will you administer?

13) A 65 kg patient diagnosed with STEMI is to receive an IV bolus dose of abciximab 0.25 mg/kg followed by a maintenance infusion of the drug at the rate of 0.125 mcg/kg/min. The abciximab is available in 5 mL vials containing 2 mg/mL.

a) How many mL will you administer for the bolus?

b) How many mcg/min will the patient receive during the maintenance infusion?

14) A 5 YO 38 lb child with a mild infection is to receive oral amoxicillin 40 mg/kg/day in divided doses every 8 hours. The amoxicillin is available in 150 mL bottles containing 250 mg/5 mL. How many mL will you administer per dose?

15) A 53 YO adult male weighing 168 lb, who is being treated for VZV encephalitis, has been prescribed acyclovir 10 mg/kg/dose IV q 8 h for 10 days. Acyclovir for injection is available in 10 and 20 mL vials containing 50 mg/mL.

a) How many mg will the patient receive each day?

b) How many mg will be patient receive each dose?

c) How many mL will the patient receive each dose?

d) How many mL will the patient receive each day?

16) A 158 lb adult male diagnosed with endocarditis has an order for gentamicin 3 mg/kg/day IV in 2 divided doses, in addition to vancomycin. The gentamicin is available in 2 mL vials containing 40 mg/mL. The facility protocol is to round the gentamicin dose to the nearest 10 mg, then calculate the volume of solution to the nearest tenth mL. How many mL will you administer per dose?

17) A 7 YO 50 lb child has been prescribed a maintenance dose of digoxin 4 mcg/kg/day PO administered in equal divided doses twice daily. Digoxin elixir is available in 60 mL bottles containing 50 mcg/mL. How many mL will you administer per dose?

18) A 4 YO 35 lb child has an order for ceftazidime 40 mg/kg IV every 8 hours. How many mg will you administer per dose?

19) Drug xyz has the following dosing guidelines:

Initiate therapy at 8-10 mg/kg/day IV once daily for 2 days, then decrease dosage by 25% for days 3 and 4, then discontinue. The prescriber has ordered an initial dose of 9 mg/kg/day for a 59 YO 182 lb male. The drug is available in 10 mL vials labeled 100 mg/mL.

a) How many mL will you administer on day 1?

b) How many mL will you administer on day 3? (Assume patient's weight has not changed.)

20) A 3 YO 31 lb child with edema has be ordered furosemide 2 mg/kg PO once daily. Furosemide oral solution is available in 60 mL bottles containing 10 mg/mL. How many mL will you administer each day?

21) A 7 YO child weighing 44 lb is diagnosed with bacterial sinusitis and is prescribed azithromycin 10 mg/kg PO once daily for 3 days. Azithromycin oral suspension is available in 15, 22.5 and 30 mL bottles containing 200 mg/5 mL. How many mL will you administer?

22) Your 67 YO 195 lb, 5 ft 10 in male patient diagnosed with testicular cancer has been prescribed ifosfamide 1200 mg/m²/day IV for 5 days. You calculate the BSA using the Mosteller method as being 2.09 m². Ifosfamide is available in 60 mL vials containing 3 g of drug. How many mL will you administer each day?

23) A 6 YO 44 lb child has been prescribed an initial loading dose of warfarin 0.2 mg/kg PO. Warfarin is available in 1 mg, 2 mg, 2.5 mg, 3 mg, 4 mg, 5 mg, 6 mg, 7.5 mg and 10 mg scored tablets.

a) How many mg will the child receive, and which tablet strength would you use?

b) On day 2, the INR comes back at 3.2 with a dosing protocol to reduce dose to 25% of the initial loading dose. How many mg would you administer, and which tablet strength would you use?

24) A 40 kg child has been prescribed an initial loading dose of warfarin 0.2 mg/kg PO. Warfarin is available in 1 mg, 2 mg, 2.5 mg, 3 mg, 4 mg, 5 mg, 6 mg, 7.5 mg and 10 mg scored tablets.

a) How many mg will the child receive, and which tablet strength would you use?

b) On day 2, the INR comes back at 2.5 with a dosing protocol to reduce dose to 50% of the initial loading dose. How many mg would you administer, and which tablet strength would you use?

25) A 42 YO adult male weighing 142 lb, who is being treated for HSE (herpes simplex encephalitis), has been prescribed acyclovir 10 mg/kg/dose IV q 8 h for 14 days. Acyclovir for injection is available in 10 and 20 mL vials containing 50 mg/mL.

a) How many mg will the patient receive each day?

b) How many mg will be patient receive each dose?

c) How many mL will the patient receive each dose?

d) How many mL will the patient receive each day?

26) Drug xyz has the following dosing guidelines:

Initiate therapy at 4-6 mg/kg/day IV once daily for 2 days, then decrease dosage by 25% for days 3 and 4, then discontinue. The prescriber has ordered an initial dose of 5 mg/kg/day IV for a 48 YO 176 lb male. The drug is available in 10 mL vials labeled 100 mg/mL.

a) How many mL will you administer on day 1?

b) How many mL will you administer on day 3? (Assume patient's weight has not changed.)

27) A 160 lb patient diagnosed with supraventricular tachycardia is to receive verapamil 5 mg IV over 2 minutes. The drug is available in 4 mL vials containing 2.5 mg/mL. How many mL will you administer?

28) A 72 YO 183 lb patient diagnosed with an M. chelonae infection has an order for amikacin 15 mg/kg IV once daily for 2 weeks (in addition to a high dose of cefoxitin). The amikacin is available in 2 mL vials containing 500 mg. How many mL will you administer each day?

29) Your 64 YO 152 lb, 5 ft 8 in female patient diagnosed with advanced bladder cancer has been prescribed ifosfamide 1500 mg/m^2/day IV for 5 days. You calculate the BSA using the Mosteller method as being 1.82 m^2. Ifosfamide is available in 60 mL vials containing 3 g of drug. How many mL will you administer each day?

30) A 16 YO is to receive cephalexin 250 mg PO q 6 h for 10 days. The drug is available in 250 mg capsules. How many capsules will the patient receive in the 10-day course of therapy?

Chapter 11
Body Surface Area Dosing Calculations

This subject was is not covered in DCFNS but will be explained here. Many drugs, especially chemotherapeutic drugs, are dosed by BSA (body surface area). The unit of measurement for BSA is square meter (m^2). While there are several formulas to calculate BSA, this book will use the Mosteller formula:

$$BSA = \sqrt{\frac{W(kg) \times H(cm)}{3600}}$$

Where BSA is in m^2, W= pt weight in kg, H = pt height in cm.

Or, if using pounds and inches:

$$BSA = \sqrt{\frac{W(lb) \times H(in)}{3131}}$$

In practice you will check with your facility on which formula to use. Also, many apps are available to quickly calculate BSA using several different formulas.

Example: Pt weight= 100 kg, height = 178 cm

$$BSA = \sqrt{\frac{100 \times 178}{3600}} = 2.22 \ m^2$$

Using the same patient, but with pounds and inches:

$$BSA = \sqrt{\frac{220 \times 70}{3131}} = 2.22 \ m^2$$

The formulas are the same for adults and children.

BSA Calculation Problems

Calculate the BSA in m² for the following individuals.

1) An adult female weighing 125 lb and 5 ft 7 in tall.

2) A 6 YO boy weighing 21 kg and 116 cm tall.

3) An adult male weighing 175 lb and 6 ft tall.

4) A 13-month-old girl weighing 21 lb and 30 in tall.

5) A 16 YO female weighing 53 kg and 161 cm tall.

6) An adult female weighing 151 lb and 5 ft 1 in tall.

7) An adult male weighing 242 lb and 6 ft 7 in tall.

8) An adult male weighing 154 lb and 5 ft 10 in tall.

9) An adult female weighing 50 kg and 4 ft 9 in tall.

10) An adult male weighing 82 kg and 183 cm tall.

Calculate the following:

11) A 49 YO male patient who weighs 170 lb and is 5 ft 11 in tall is being treated for refractory multiple myeloma and will be placed on a carfilzomib 20/27 mg/m² IV twice weekly regimen. Cycle 1 of the regimen will be 20 mg/m² infused over 10 minutes on days 1 and 2, followed by 27 mg/m² over 10 minutes on days 8, 9, 15, and 16 of a 28-day treatment cycle.

a) Calculate the patient's BSA.

b) Calculate the dose in mg the patient will receive on days 1 and 2.

c) Calculate the dose the patient will receive on days 8, 9, 15, and 16.

12) A 68 YO male patient who weighs 155 lb and is 5 ft 9 in tall is being treated for acute myeloid leukemia with IV idarubicin 12 mg/m²/day for 3 days (in combination with cytarabine).

a) Calculate the patient's BSA.

b) Calculate the daily dose in mg for this patient.

13) A 9 YO 64 lb boy who is 4 ft 5 in tall is to receive IV topotecan 2.4 mg/m² once daily for 7 days for treatment of acute lymphoblastic leukemia.

a) Calculate the patient's BSA.

b) Calculate the daily dose in mg for this patient.

14) A 10 YO male child who weighs 32 kg and is 139 cm tall will start the BEACOPP regimen for treatment of Hodgkin lymphoma. Oral prednisone is part of the regimen dosed at 40 mg/m²/day in 2 divided doses on days 0 to 13.

a) Calculate the patient's BSA.

b) How many milligrams of prednisone will the patient receive per dose?

Chapter 12
Pediatric Dosing Problems

The recommended oral dosage of cephalexin to treat impetigo in infants, children and adolescents is 25 to 50 mg/kg/day divided every 6 to 8 hours (with a maximum dose of 250 mg/dose) for at least 7 days. A 15-month-old, 23 lb child has been prescribed 100 mg PO q 8 h for 7 days. The drug is available as 250 mg/5 mL.

1) What is the recommended range in mg/dose for this child when dosed q 8 h?

2) Is the prescribed dosage within the recommended range for impetigo?

3) What is the range in mL/dose for this child?

4) How many mL/dose would the child receive for the prescribed dosage?

The recommended oral dosage of amoxicillin to treat acute otitis media (AOM) for infants (2 months and over) and children is 80 to 90 mg/kg/day in divided doses every 12 hours. The duration of therapy will vary with patient age and severity of symptoms. A 6-month-old infant weighing 18 lb has been prescribed 350 mg q 12 h. The drug is available as 250 mg/5 mL.

5) What is the recommended range in mg/dose for this child?

6) Is the prescribed dosage within the recommended range for AOM?

7) What is the recommended range in mL/dose for this child?

8) How many mL/dose would the child receive for the prescribed dosage?

The recommended oral dosage for diphenhydramine is 5 mg/kg/day divided into 3-4 doses when treating allergies in infants, children and adolescents. A 6 YO 46 lb male child has been prescribed 25 mg PO q 6 h. Diphenhydramine is available as an oral solution containing 12.5 mg/5 mL.

9) Is this a reasonable dosage for this child?

10) How many mL/dose will the child receive?

Azithromycin has several different oral regimens to treat OM in children six months and older. The 3-day regimen is 10 mg/kg once daily for 3 days (maximum: 500 mg/day). Azithromycin is available as 200 mg/5 mL.

11) How many mL will a 3 YO boy weighing 31 lb receive each day?

The dosing guidelines for oral morphine sulfate solution for treating moderate to severe acute pain in infants >6 months, children and adolescents who are <50 kg is 0.2 to 0.5 mg/kg/dose every 3 to 4 hours as needed and for children and adolescents 50 kg and over it is 15 to 20 mg every 3 to 4 hours as needed. Morphine sulfate oral solution 2 mg/mL and 4 mg/mL is available.

12) Using the above information, what is the normal mg/dose range for a 7 YO 23 kg male child?

13) What is the normal mL/dose range using the 2 mg/mL solution for a 15-month-old 23 lb child?

14) The prescriber has ordered 2 mL/dose of the 4 mg/mL morphine sulfate solution for your 4 YO patient who weighs 17 kg. Is this dose within the dosing guidelines?

15) The prescriber, who wants to order the highest recommended dose of oral morphine sulfate solution for a 14 kg 3 YO child, has ordered 3.9 mL of the 4 mg/mL solution. Is this the correct dose? If not, what is a possible cause of the error?

The general dosing guidelines for IV ampicillin in treating mild to moderate infections in infants, children and adolescents is 100 to 150 mg/kg/day divided every 6 hours with a maximum daily dose of 4000 mg. Using this information, answer the following questions.

16) What is the mg/dose range for a 9 YO 63 lb male child?

17) What is the mg/day range for a 6 YO 20 kg female child?

18) The health care provider ordered 700 mg IV q 6 h for a 50 lb 7 YO female child.

a) Is this dosage within the general dosing guidelines?

b) How many mg/kg/day will this child be receiving?

19) A 32 kg 10 YO female has been prescribed a dosage 140 mg/kg/day divided every 6 hours. Does this dosage fall within the general dosing guidelines?

Chapter 13
Pediatric Maintenance Fluid Replacement Calculations

Weight	24 Hour Fluid Requirement
Infants 3.5 to 10 kg	100 mL/kg
Children 11-20 kg	1000 mL + 50 mL/kg for every kg over 10
For children > 20 kg	1500 mL + 20 mL/kg for every kg over 20, up to a maximum of 2400 mL daily.

Use the above table in the following calculations. Round to the nearest mL and nearest mL/h.

Example: Calculate the daily maintenance fluid requirement for an NPO child weighing 12 kg.

1000 mL + 2 kg (50 mL/kg) = 1000 mL + 100 mL = 1100 mL

At what rate would you set the infusion pump?

1100 mL/24 h = 46 mL/h

1) Calculate the daily maintenance fluid requirement for an NPO child weighing 14 kg.

2) Calculate the daily maintenance fluid requirement for an NPO child weighing 23 kg.

3) Calculate the daily maintenance fluid requirement for an NPO child weighing 8.5 kg.

4) Calculate the daily maintenance fluid requirement for an NPO child weighing 41.5 kg.

5) Calculate the infusion rate to the nearest mL/h to deliver daily maintenance fluids to an NPO child weighing 32 kg.

6) A 35 kg NPO child is on 70% fluid maintenance (70% of the calculated amount in the above table). At what rate will you set the infusion pump?

7) What is the daily maintenance fluid requirement for an NPO child on 70% fluid maintenance who weighs 45 kg? At what rate will you set the infusion pump?

8) What is the daily maintenance fluid requirement for an NPO child on 70% fluid maintenance who weighs 19.5 kg? At what rate will you set the infusion pump?

9) At what rate will you set the infusion pump to deliver maintenance fluids to a 15 kg NPO child who is on 70% fluid maintenance?

10) Calculate the daily maintenance fluid requirement for an NPO child weighing 28 kg.

11) What is the daily maintenance fluid requirement for an NPO child on 70% fluid maintenance who weighs 36 kg?

12) Calculate the daily maintenance fluid requirement for an NPO child weighing 31.5 kg.

Unit 4: IV Flow Rate Calculations

Chapter 14: IV Flow Rate Calculations Level I
Corresponding Chapter and pages in DCFNS: Chapter 10, pp. 39-43.
Importance: 10/10. These problems start you off with easy mL/h, gtts/min and volume infused problems. If you have followed DCFNS, you will understand that these problems are set up the same general way that unit conversion and dosage problems are.

Chapter 15: IV Flow Rate Calculations Level 2
Corresponding Chapter and pages in DCFNS: Chapter 10, pp. 39-43.
Importance: 10/10. Although DCFNS only had a few advanced problems, it provided the basic knowledge on how to set up and solve these problems. You can choose to work all 40 of these problems, or just a few. The important thing is that you understand there is a foolproof, step by step approach to these problems which doesn't involve memorizing any formulas.

Chapter 16: IV Flow Rate Adjustments
Corresponding Chapter and pages in DCFNS: None. New material for this book.
Importance: 10/10. These situations will arise in real life and you should know how to handle them.

Chapter 17: Heparin Infusion Calculations
Corresponding Chapter and pages in DCFNS: None. New material for this book.
Importance: 8/10. This chapter as added to give an example of one of the many drugs which require close monitoring and adjustment per protocol. The odds that you will be presented with heparin dosing calculations which exactly match the protocol in this book are slim, but you should understand the general procedure.

Chapter 14
IV Flow Rate Calculations Level I

Round all drops/min calculations to the nearest drop and all mL/h calculations to the nearest tenth mL/h.

Calculate the flow rate in mL/h.

1) 1000 mL infused over 4 hours.

2) 500 mL infused over 6 hours.

3) 1000 mL infused over 8 hours.

4) 500 mL infused over 3 hours.

5) 1000 mL infused over 5 hours.

6) 250 mL infused over 90 minutes.

7) 500 mL infused over 4 hours 15 minutes.

8) 1000 mL infused over 6 hours 30 minutes.

9) 250 mL infused over 45 minutes.

10) 500 mL infused over 3 hours 15 minutes.

Calculate the flow rate in drops/min.

11) 1000 mL infused over 5 hours with a drop factor of 20 (20 gtts/mL).

12) 1000 mL infused over 6 hours with a drop factor of 15 (15 gtts/mL).

13) 250 mL infused over 2 hours with a microdrip set (60 gtts/mL).

14) 500 mL infused over 7 hours with a drop factor of 10.

15) 100 mL infused over 1 h with a drop factor of 15.

16) 500 mL infused over 4 hours with a drop factor of 20.

17) 500 mL infused over 90 minutes with a drop factor of 10.

18) 1000 mL infused over 3 hours 30 minutes with a drop factor of 15.

19) 1000 mL infused over 10 hours 15 minutes with a drop factor of 60.

20) 750 mL infused over 4 hours 20 minutes with a drop factor of 15.

Calculate the length of time in hours and minutes, rounded to the nearest minute, required to infuse the following:

21) 1000 mL at 90 mL/h.

22) 500 mL at 125 mL/h.

23) 100 mL at 64 mL/h.

24) 250 mL at 31 gtts/min with a drop factor of 20.

25) 500 mL at 43 gtts/min with a drop factor of 10.

26) 1000 mL at 50 gtts/min with a drop factor of 15.

27) 500 mL at 24 gtts/min with a drop factor of 20.

28) 1000 mL at 60 gtts/min with a drop factor of 10.

29) 500 mL at 25 mL/h.

30) 1000 mL at 60 mL/h.

Calculate the volume infused in the following scenarios. Round to the nearest mL.

31) Infusion rate of 40 mL/h for 3 hours 15 min.

32) Infusion rate of 65 mL/h for 2 hours 30 min.

33) Infusion rate of 24 gtts/min, drop factor 20, for 4 hours 20 min.

34) Infusion rate of 72 gtts/min, drop factor 15, for 6 hours 15 min.

35) Infusion rate of 32 mL/h for 3 h 10 minutes.

36) Infusion rate of 45 gtts/min, drop factor 20, for 6 hours 15 min.

37) Infusion rate of 30 mL per hour for 4 hours 30 min.

38) Infusion rate of 62 mL per hour for 1 hour 15 min.

39) Infusion rate of 34 mL/h for 90 min.

40) Infusion rate of 45 gtts/min, drop factor 20, for 6 hours 20 min.

Chapter 15
IV Flow Rate Calculations Level 2

Round all drops/min to the nearest drop. Round all mL/hour rates for the infusion pump to the nearest tenth mL/hour.

1) A healthcare provider has ordered dobutamine 10 mcg/kg/min IV for your 68 YO patient who weighs 172 lb. The dobutamine is available as 1000 mg/250 mL. At what rate will you set the IV infusion pump?

2) Mrs. Robinson, who has been diagnosed with acute decompensated heart failure, has an order for nitroglycerin 10 mcg/min IV. Mrs. Robinson weighs 142 lb. The NTG is available as 100 mg/250 mL. At what rate will you set the IV infusion pump?

3) A 170 lb patient has an order for dopamine 15 mcg/kg/min to treat heart failure. The courteous pharmacy staff sends a 250 mL bag labeled dopamine 3200 mcg/mL. At what rate will you set the IV infusion pump?

4) Your 81 kg patient has an order for dobutamine 15 mcg/kg/min IV to start at 0900. The dobutamine is available as 500 mg in 250 mL D5W. At what rate will you set the IV infusion pump?

5) Your 67 YO 74 kg patient has an order for a lidocaine infusion at the rate of 20 mcg/kg/min. You have a 250 mL bag labeled "Lidocaine HCl and 5% Dextrose Injection USP". Lidocaine 2 g (8 mg/mL) is printed in big red letters in the middle of the label. What rate will you set the IV infusion pump?

6) Your 71 kg patient is receiving a dopamine infusion at the rate of 14 mL/h. The dopamine is mixed as 200 mg of dopamine in 250 mL of D5W. The infusion has been running for 1 hour 45 minutes. How many mcg/kg/min is the patient receiving?

7) A 38 YO female weighing 125 lb, who is being treated for a bite wound infection, has an order for ciprofloxacin 400 mg IV every 12 hours to be infused by slow IV infusion over 60 minutes. Ciprofloxacin is available in 200 mL bags containing 400 mg. You are using an IV administration set with a drop factor of 20. How many drops/min will you administer?

8) Your 140 lb, 5 ft 4 in female patient has an order for dobutamine 5 mcg/kg/min IV to start at 1400. The dobutamine is available as 1000 mcg/mL. At what rate will you set the IV infusion pump?

9) Your 180 lb patient in vasodilatory shock has been ordered vasopressin 0.03 units/min IV. The vasopressin is available as 20 units/100 mL. At what rate will you set the IV infusion pump?

10) A physician has ordered dobutamine 4 mcg/kg/min IV for your 57 YO patient who weighs 75 kg. The dobutamine is available as 1000 mg in 250 mL D5W. At what rate will you set the IV infusion pump?

11) A 52 YO female who weighs 76 kg is to receive vancomycin 2 g in 400 mL D5W at a rate of 10 mg/min. At what rate will you set the IV infusion pump?

12) A 57 YO male weighing 165 lb, who has been diagnosed with meningitis, has an order for gentamicin 5 mg/kg/day in 3 divided doses. Each dose is to be administered over 120 minutes. The drug is available in 100 mL bags containing 125 mg. At what rate will you set the IV infusion pump?

13) Mr. Dombroski, who has been diagnosed with acute decompensated heart failure, has an order for nitroglycerin 15 mcg/min IV. Mr. Dombroski weighs 195 lb and is 6 ft 1 in tall. The NTG is available as 100 mg/250 mL. At what rate will you set the IV infusion pump?

14) Your 55 kg patient is experiencing angina and has an order for nitroglycerin 5 mcg/min IV. The NTG is available as 100 mg/250 mL. At what rate will you set the IV infusion pump?

15) You are starting your 174 lb patient on a lidocaine infusion at the rate of 20 mcg/kg/min. You have a 500 mL bag labeled "Lidocaine HCl and 5% Dextrose Injection USP". Lidocaine 2 g (4 mg/mL) is printed in big red letters in the middle of the label. What rate will you set the IV infusion pump?

16) A 21 lb, 10-month-old infant, in shock has an order for norepinephrine 0.1 mcg/kg/min IV. The norepinephrine is available in a concentration of 8 mcg/mL. At what rate will you set the IV infusion pump?

17) Your 55 YO female patient, who has been diagnosed with septic shock, weighs 155 lb. She has an order for norepinephrine 0.1 mcg/kg/min IV. The pharmacy delivers a bag containing 4 mg norepinephrine in 250 mL D5NS. At what rate will you set the IV infusion pump?

18) A 55 YO male weighing 60 kg is to receive tobramycin 2 mg/kg/dose IV every 8 hours for a severe infection. Each dose will be administered over 40 minutes.

a) How many mg will the patient receive each dose?

b) The pharmacy sends over the appropriate dose of tobramycin in a 100 mL bag of NS. At what rate will you set the IV infusion pump?

19) Your 130 lb female patient has an order for dobutamine 5 mcg/kg/min IV to start at 1200. The dobutamine is available as 1000 mcg/mL. At what rate will you set the IV infusion pump?

20) A patient who weighs 175 lb is suffering from acute hypertension and has an order to start an infusion of nitroprusside 0.4 mcg/kg/min. The pharmacy delivers a 1000 mL bag containing 50 mg nitroprusside in D5W. At what rate will you set the IV infusion pump?

21) A 190 lb patient is receiving a 4 mg/mL lidocaine infusion at the rate of 24 mL/h. How many mcg/kg/min is the patient receiving?

22) Your 95 kg patient is receiving a dopamine infusion at the rate of 15 mL/h. The dopamine is mixed as 200 mg of dopamine in 250 mL of D5W. The infusion has been running for 1 hour 25 minutes. How many mcg/kg/min is the patient receiving?

23) Your 60 kg patient has an order for dobutamine 10 mcg/kg/min IV to start at 1100. The dobutamine is available as 500 mg in 250 mL D5W. At what rate will you set the IV infusion pump?

24) Your 160 lb patient in vasodilatory shock has had his vasopressin titrated up to 0.035 units/min IV. The vasopressin is available as 20 units/100 mL. What rate will you set the IV infusion pump?

25) Your 65 kg patient in septic shock has been ordered norepinephrine 1.5 mcg/kg/min IV. The norepinephrine is available as 4 mg in 250 mL D5W. What rate will you set the IV infusion pump?

26) A 77 kg patient is receiving a 4 mg/mL lidocaine infusion at the rate of 18 mL/h. How many mcg/kg/min is the patient receiving?

27) A 9 kg, 8-month-old infant, in shock has an order for norepinephrine 0.05 mcg/kg/min IV. The norepinephrine is available in a concentration of 8 mcg/mL. At what rate will you set the IV infusion pump?

28) A 49 YO male who weighs 45 kg is to receive IV vancomycin 1 g in 200 mL D5W at a rate of 10 mg/min. At what rate will you set the IV infusion pump?

29) A 67 YO male weighing 80 kg, who has been diagnosed with endocarditis, has an order for gentamicin 3 mg/kg/day in 2 divided doses. Each dose is to be administered over 120 minutes. The drug is available in 100 mL bags containing 120 mg. At what rate will you set the IV infusion pump?

30) Your 142 lb patient is experiencing angina and has had his IV nitroglycerin titrated up to 15 mcg/min. The NTG is available as 100 mg/250 mL. At what rate will you set the IV infusion pump?

31) A 38 YO female weighing 125 lb, who is being treated for a bite wound infection, has an order for ciprofloxacin 400 mg IV every 12 hours to be infused by slow IV infusion over 60 minutes. Ciprofloxacin is available in 200 mL bags containing 400 mg. You are using an IV administration set with a drop factor of 10. How many drops/min will you administer?

32) An 84 kg patient has an order for dopamine 10 mcg/kg/min IV to treat cardiogenic shock. The pharmacy sends a 500 mL bag labeled dopamine 1600 mcg/mL. At what rate will you set the IV infusion pump?

33) Your 45 YO female patient, who has been diagnosed with septic shock, weighs 67 kg. She has an order for norepinephrine 0.1 mcg/kg/min IV. The pharmacy delivers a bag containing 4 mg norepinephrine in 250 mL D5NS. At what rate will you set the IV infusion pump?

34) H.M., a 70 YO female weighing 68 kg with heart failure, has an order for a continuous IV infusion of milrinone 0.5 mcg/kg/min. Milrinone is available in 100 mL bags containing 20 mg. At what rate will you set the IV infusion pump?

35) Your 65 kg 68 YO patient, diagnosed with bradycardia, has an order for epinephrine 0.4 mcg/kg/min. The pharmacy sends over a bag containing 1 mg epinephrine in 250 mL NS. At what rate will you set the IV infusion pump?

36) A patient who weighs 74 kg is suffering from acute hypertension and has an order to start an infusion of nitroprusside 0.5 mcg/kg/min. The pharmacy delivers a 1000 mL bag containing 50 mg nitroprusside in D5W. At what rate will you set the IV infusion pump?

37) A 45 YO male weighing 65 kg is to receive tobramycin 2.5 mg/kg/dose IV every 12 hours for a severe infection. Each dose will be administered over 60 minutes.

a) How many mg will the patient receive each dose?

b) The pharmacy sends over the appropriate dose of tobramycin in a 100 mL bag of NS. At what rate will you set the IV infusion pump?

38) Your 64 kg patient in septic shock has been ordered norepinephrine 2 mcg/kg/min IV. The norepinephrine is available as 4 mg in 250 mL D5W. What rate will you set the IV infusion pump?

39) J.W., a 70 YO male weighing 75 kg with heart failure has an order for a continuous IV infusion of milrinone 0.6 mcg/kg/min. Milrinone is available in 100 mL bags containing 20 mg. At what rate will you set the IV infusion pump?

40) Your 55 kg 62 YO patient diagnosed with bradycardia has an order for epinephrine 0.3 mcg/kg/min. The efficient pharmacy sends over a bag containing 1 mg epinephrine in 250 mL NS. At what rate will you set the IV infusion pump?

Chapter 16
IV Flow Rate Adjustments

Occasionally, you will be required to adjust the flow rate of an IV which hasn't been infusing at the desired rate. For example, you may have an order to infuse a 1000 mL bag over 8 hours, but after 4 hours you notice that 600 mL remain, meaning that only 400 mL has infused. You must now recalculate the flow rate so that the remaining 600 mL infuses over 4 hours. Depending on facility policy, you may have to contact the prescriber if a significant adjustment has been made. For purposes of these problems, assume the prescriber must be contacted for any flow rate change of 25% or more.

Example: A 1000 mL bag of D5W was started at 0900 and set to infuse over 6 hours with a drop factor of 20. At 1100 you monitor the infusion and notice that 800 mL remains.

What is the initial calculated rate in gtts/min?

$$\frac{1000 \text{ mL}}{6 \text{ h}} \left(\frac{20 \text{ gtt}}{\text{mL}}\right)\left(\frac{1 \text{ h}}{60 \text{ min}}\right) = \frac{56 \text{ gtt}}{\text{min}}$$

What will be the new rate in gtts/min?

You will infuse the remaining 800 mL over 4 hours using the same drop set.

$$\frac{800 \text{ mL}}{4 \text{ h}} \left(\frac{20 \text{ gtt}}{\text{mL}}\right)\left(\frac{1 \text{ h}}{60 \text{ min}}\right) = \frac{67 \text{ gtt}}{\text{min}}$$

What is the percent change?

The formula to calculate percent change is:

$$\frac{\text{Final} - \text{Initial}}{\text{Initial}} (100\%) = \% \text{ Change}$$

All the units will cancel, so we can just use 67 and 56, rather than 67 gtts/min and 56 gtts/min.

$$\frac{67 - 56}{56} (100\%) = 19.6 \%$$

Will you contact the prescriber?

No, 19.6% is <25%.

You have an order for a 500 mL bag of NS to infuse over 4 hours with a drop factor of 10. The bag was started at 1700. At 1800 you notice that 300 mL remain.

1) What is the initial calculated rate in gtts/min?

2) What will be the new rate in gtts/min?

3) What is the percent change?

4) Will you contact the prescriber?

You have an order for a 1000 mL bag of NS to infuse over 3 hours with a drop factor of 15. The bag was started at 0600. At 0700 you notice that 750 mL remain.

5) What is the initial calculated rate in gtts/min?

6) What will be the new rate in gtts/min?

7) What is the percent change?

8) Will you contact the prescriber?

You have an order for a 1000 mL bag of D5W to infuse over 12 hours with a drop factor of 20. The bag was started at 0800. At 1400 you notice that 625 mL remain.

9) What is the initial calculated rate in gtts/min?

10) What will be the new rate in gtts/min?

11) What is the percent change?

12) Will you contact the prescriber?

You have an order for a 500 mL bag of NS to infuse over 2 hours with a drop factor of 10. The bag was started at 1100. At 1130 you notice that 450 mL remain.

13) What is the initial calculated rate in gtts/min?

14) What will be the new rate in gtts/min?

15) What is the percent change?

16) Will you contact the prescriber?

You have an order for a 250 mL bag of NS to infuse over 2 hours with a drop factor of 60. The bag was started at 2100. At 2130 you notice that 150 mL remain.

17) What is the initial calculated rate in gtts/min?

18) What will be the new rate in gtts/min?

19) What is the percent change?

20) Will you contact the prescriber?

You have an order for a 1000 mL bag of D5W to infuse over 5 hours with a drop factor of 15. The bag was started at 0800. Two hours later you notice that 700 mL remain.

21) What is the initial calculated rate in gtts/min?

22) What will be the new rate in gtts/min?

23) What is the percent change?

24) Will you contact the prescriber?

You have an order for a 500 mL bag of NS to infuse over 4 hours with a drop factor of 15. The bag was started at 0100. At 0300 you notice that 150 mL remain.

25) What is the initial calculated rate in gtts/min?

26) What will be the new rate in gtts/min?

27) What is the percent change?

28) Will you contact the prescriber?

You have an order for a 1000 mL bag of NS to infuse over 9 hours with a drop factor of 10. The bag was started at 1600. At 1800 you notice that 450 mL remain.

29) What is the initial calculated rate in gtts/min?

30) What will be the new rate in gtts/min?

31) What is the percent change?

32) Will you contact the prescriber?

You have an order for a 500 mL bag of NS to infuse over 2 hours with a drop factor of 15. The bag was started at 1600. At 1700 you notice that 400 mL remain.

33) What is the initial calculated rate in gtts/min?

34) What will be the new rate in gtts/min?

35) What is the percent change?

36) Will you contact the prescriber?

You have an order for a 500 mL bag of NS to infuse over 7 hours with a drop factor of 20. The bag was started at 1900. At 2000 you notice that 300 mL remain.

37) What is the initial calculated rate in gtts/min?

38) What will be the new rate in gtts/min?

39) What is the percent change?

40) Will you contact the prescriber?

Chapter 17
Heparin Infusion and Adjustment Calculations

Heparin is an anticoagulant used to treat various conditions including heart attacks, deep vein thrombosis, atrial fibrillation, and pulmonary embolism. Heparin infusion protocols vary by facility, so these practice problems will probably differ from your actual calculations.

For this set of problems, use the following information:

- Round bolus doses to the nearest 500 units.
- Round infusion doses to the nearest 100 units/h.
- Use 25,000 units heparin/250 mL D5W (100 units/mL) for infusions.
- Use 5000 units/mL for IVP bolus calculations.
- Heparin levels are monitored by anti-Xa assay 6 hours after starting the infusion and 6 hours after each dosage adjustment.
- After two consecutive anti-Xa levels are within therapeutic range (0.3-0.7 units/mL) decrease to daily monitoring.
- Call prescriber if two consecutive anti-Xa levels are > 0.9 or < 0.2.
- Use the following table for dosage adjustments.

Anti-Xa (units/mL)	Re-Bolus	Hold Infusion	Dosage Adjustment
< 0.2	80 units/kg	No	Increase 4 units/kg/h
0.2-0.29	40 units/kg	No	Increase 2 units/kg/h
0.3-0.7	No	No	No Change
0.71-0.8	No	No	Decrease 1 unit/kg/h
0.81-0.9	No	30 min	Decrease 2 units/kg/h
>0.9	No	60 min	Decrease 3 units/kg/h

Pt A.K., who weighs 190 lb, has been admitted with a diagnosis of DVT and has the following heparin order:
Initial bolus: 80 units/kg (max 10,000 units)
Initial infusion: 18 units/kg/h (initial max of 1800 units/h)

1) Calculate the bolus dose in units.

2) Calculate the bolus dose in mL.

3) Calculate the initial infusion rate in units/h.

4) Calculate the initial infusion rate in mL/h.

5) The initial infusion was started at 1300. At 1900 you order an anti-Xa assay and it comes back at 0.75 units/mL. What will the new infusion rate be in units/h?

6) At 0100 the following day another anti-Xa assay is ordered and comes back at 0.69 units/mL. Will you, or the on-duty nurse, adjust the dose? If so, what will the new infusion rate be in units/h?

7) At 0700 another anti-Xa assay is ordered which comes back at 0.70 units/mL. What do you do?

Pt B.J., who weighs 194 lb, has been admitted with a diagnosis of unstable angina and has the following heparin order:
Initial bolus: 60 units/kg (max 5,000 units)
Initial infusion: 12 units/kg/h (initial max of 1000 units/h)
8) Calculate the bolus dose in units.

9) Calculate the bolus dose in mL.

10) Calculate the initial infusion rate in units/h.

11) Calculate the initial infusion rate in mL/h.

12) The initial infusion was started at 1400. At 2000 you order an anti-Xa assay and it comes back at 0.25 units/mL. What course of action will you take? Include all calculations.

13) At 0200 the following day another anti-Xa assay is ordered and comes back at 0.51 units/mL. Will you, or the on-duty nurse, adjust the dose? If so, what will the new infusion rate be in units/h?

14) At 0800 another anti-Xa assay is ordered which comes back at 0.72 units/mL. What do you do?

Pt A.R., a 45 YO female weighing 135 lb, has been admitted with a diagnosis of PE and has the following heparin order:
Initial bolus: 80 units/kg (max 10,000 units)
Initial infusion: 18 units/kg/h (initial max of 1800 units/h)
15) Calculate the bolus dose in units.

16) Calculate the bolus dose in mL.

17) Calculate the initial infusion rate in units/h.

18) Calculate the initial infusion rate in mL/h.

19) The initial infusion was started at 0930. At 3:30 PM you order an anti-Xa assay and it comes back at 0.95 units/mL. What course of action will you take? What will the new infusion rate be in units/h?

20) At 2130 another anti-Xa assay is ordered and comes back at 0.91 units/mL. What is your course of action?

21) After contacting the prescriber after the second anti-Xa assay >9.0, you are instructed to decrease the dosage by 3 units/kg/h. What will be the new rate in units/h?

Pt J.W., who weighs 74 kg, has been admitted with a diagnosis of stroke and has the following heparin order:
Initial bolus: None
Initial infusion: 12 units/kg/h (initial max of 1200 units/h)
22) Calculate the bolus dose in units.

23) Calculate the bolus dose in mL.

24) Calculate the initial infusion rate in units/h.

25) Calculate the initial infusion rate in mL/h.

26) The initial infusion was started at 6:30 AM. At 12:30 PM you order an anti-Xa assay and it comes back at 0.53 units/mL. What will the new infusion rate be in units/h?

27) At 6:30 PM another anti-Xa assay is ordered and comes back at 0.51 units/mL. Will you, or the on-duty nurse, adjust the dose? If so, what will the new infusion rate be in mL/h?

28) At 0700 another anti-Xa assay is ordered which comes back at 0.53 units/mL. What do you do? When will you order the next anti-Xa?

Pt T.G., who weighs 86 kg, has been admitted with a diagnosis of DVT and has the following heparin order:
Initial bolus: 80 units/kg (max 10,000 units)
Initial infusion: 18 units/kg/h (initial max of 1800 units/h)

29) Calculate the bolus dose in units.

30) Calculate the bolus dose in mL.

31) Calculate the initial infusion rate in units/h.

32) Calculate the initial infusion rate in mL/h.

33) The initial infusion was started at 1300. At 1900 you order an anti-Xa assay and it comes back at 0.75 units/mL. What will the new infusion rate be in units/h?

34) At 0100 the following day another anti-Xa assay is ordered and comes back at 0.69 units/mL. Will you, or the on-duty nurse, adjust the dose? If so, what will the new infusion rate be in units/h?

35) At 0700 another anti-Xa assay is ordered which comes back at 0.70 units/mL. What do you do?

Pt M.J., who weighs 109 kg, has been admitted with a diagnosis of DVT and has the following heparin order:
Initial bolus: 80 units/kg (max 10,000 units)
Initial infusion: 18 units/kg/h (initial max of 1800 units/h)

36) Calculate the bolus dose in units.

37) Calculate the bolus dose in mL.

38) Calculate the initial infusion rate in units/h.

39) Calculate the initial infusion rate in mL/h.

40) The initial infusion was started at 1015. At 1615 you order an anti-Xa assay and it comes back at 0.24 units/mL. What is your course of action? Show all calculations.

41) At 2215 another anti-Xa assay is ordered and comes back at 0.41 units/mL. Will you, or the on-duty nurse, adjust the dose? If so, what will the new infusion rate be in units/h?

42) At 0415 another anti-Xa assay is ordered which comes back at 0.45 units/mL. What do you do?

Pt T.W., who weighs 69 kg, has been admitted with a diagnosis of DVT and has the following heparin order:
Initial bolus: 80 units/kg (max 10,000 units)
Initial infusion: 18 units/kg/h (initial max of 1800 units/h)

43) Calculate the bolus dose in units.

44) Calculate the bolus dose in mL.

45) Calculate the initial infusion rate in units/h.

46) Calculate the initial infusion rate in mL/h.

47) The initial infusion was started at 0600. At 1200 you order an anti-Xa assay and it comes back at 0.82 units/mL. What is your course of action? What will the new infusion rate be in units/h?

48) At 1800 another anti-Xa assay is ordered and comes back at 0.74 units/mL. Will you, or the on-duty nurse, adjust the dose? If so, what will the new infusion rate be in units/h?

49) At 0000 another anti-Xa assay is ordered which comes back at 0.71 units/mL. What do you do? If you adjust the dosage, what is the new rate in mL/h?

Pt W.W., who weighs 46 kg, has been admitted with a diagnosis of PE and has the following heparin order:
Initial bolus: 80 units/kg (max 10,000 units)
Initial infusion: 18 units/kg/h (initial max of 1800 units/h)
50) Calculate the bolus dose in units.

51) Calculate the bolus dose in mL.

52) Calculate the initial infusion rate in units/h.

53) Calculate the initial infusion rate in mL/h.

54) The initial infusion was started at 1100. At 1700 you order an anti-Xa assay and it comes back at 0.22 units/mL. What course of action do you take? Show calculations.

55) At 2300 another anti-Xa assay is ordered and comes back at 0.40 units/mL. Will you, or the on-duty nurse, adjust the dose? If so, what will the new infusion rate be in units/h?

56) At 0500 the next day, another anti-Xa assay is ordered which comes back at 0.42 units/mL. What do you do?

Pt J.J., a 72 YO male weighing 85 kg has been admitted with a diagnosis of unstable angina and has the following heparin order:
Initial bolus: 60 units/kg (max 5,000 units)
Initial infusion: 12 units/kg/h (initial max of 1000 units/h)

57) Calculate the bolus dose in units.

58) Calculate the bolus dose in mL.

59) Calculate the initial infusion rate in units/h.

60) Calculate the initial infusion rate in mL/h.

61) The initial infusion was started at 1600. At 2200 you order an anti-Xa assay and it comes back at 0.82 units/mL. What course of action will you take? Include all calculations.

62) At 0400 the following day another anti-Xa assay is ordered and comes back at 0.75 units/mL. Will you, or the on-duty nurse, adjust the dose? If so, what will the new infusion rate be in units/h?

63) At 1000 another anti-Xa assay is ordered which comes back at 0.71 units/mL. What do you do?

Unit 5: Percent and Ratio Strength Calculations

Chapter 18: Percent
Corresponding Chapter and pages in DCFNS: Chapter 11, pp. 44-45.
Importance: 10/10. You must know the basics of percent problems, not only for nursing school, but also for everyday life.

Chapter 19: Percent Strength
Corresponding Chapter and pages in DCFNS: Chapter 11, pp. 48-50.
Importance: 7/10. You will deal with solutions everyday which are labeled in percent strength (D5W, NS, etc.) and should know what it means. Your dosage calculations tests probably won't emphasize these problems, but there might be a few. It is easy to learn, so go for it.

Chapter 20: Percent Change
Corresponding Chapter and pages in DCFNS: Chapter 11, p. 47.
Importance: 8/10. Nursing dosage calculations exams will frequently include these types of problems. They are easy and should be learned. There are also a lot of everyday uses for these calculations.

Chapter 21: Ratio Strength
Corresponding Chapter and pages in DCFNS: Chapter 11, pp. 51-52.
Importance: 7/10. Ratio strength labeling of single entity drugs is being discontinued, but you may still encounter them. What to know: They are dangerous and look on the vial for the mg/mL concentration when doing calculations. You can do a few problems just to boost your confidence.

Chapter 18
Percent

Convert the following numbers to percents.

Problem	Number	Percent
Example	0.37	0.37 (100%) = 37%
1	0.21	
2	0.88	
3	2.38	
4	3.89	
5	0.005	
6	0.02	
7	1.35	
8	0.41	
9	0.69	
10	7.55	

Convert the following percents to numbers.

Problem	Percent	Number
Example	32%	32%/100% = 0.32
11	42.5%	
12	89%	
13	1.1%	
14	64.3%	
15	5.6%	
16	4.35%	
17	3.9%	
18	5.2%	
19	1.7%	
20	0.3%	

Chapter 19
Percent Strength

Express the following as percent strength solutions and include the type of solution (w/w, w/v, v/v, v/w).

1) 2.45 g NaCl in 2 L

2) 1 g HC in 200 g HC ointment

3) 10 g urea in 40 g urea ointment

4) 20 mL ETOH in 100 mL ETOH solution

5) 2.5 mg betamethasone in 10 g betamethasone ointment

6) 25 mcg NaCl in 0.25 mL

7) 510 mg NaHCO$_3$ in 200 mL

8) 7.5 g NaCl in 1000 mL

9) 5 g KCl in 200 mL

10) 10 g salicylic acid in 200 g salicylic acid cream

Answer the following:

11) How many mg of bupivacaine are in 45 mL of 0.5% bupivacaine solution?

12) How many mg of NaCl are in 60 mL of 0.9% NaCl (normal saline)?

13) How many mg of lidocaine are in 250 mL of 1% lidocaine?

14) How many g of KCl are in 473 mL of 10% KCl?

15) How many mcg of dextrose are in 1 drop of 5% dextrose solution if there are 20 drops/mL?

16) How many g of NaCl are in 1.5 L of NS (normal saline-0.9% NaCl)?

17) How many mg of triamcinolone are in 60 g of 0.1% triamcinolone ointment?

18) How many g of HC are in 200 g of 2.5% HC ointment?

19) How many mcg of fluocinolone are in 50 g of 0.01% fluocinolone cream?

20) How many grams of dextrose are in 2 L of D5W (5% dextrose in water)?

Chapter 20
Percent Change

- The formula to calculate percent change is:

$$\frac{\text{Final} - \text{Initial}}{\text{Initial}} (100\%) = \% \text{ Change}$$

- Remember, the percent change can be positive or negative.
- If the units are the same, they will cancel out and there is no need to include them in the calculations.

Calculate the percent change in the following scenarios. Round to the nearest tenth percent.

1) Your patient weighed 86 kg on admission and weighs 82 kg today.

2) Your patient weighed 194 lb on admission and weighs 197 lb today.

3) A patient's daily dose of a drug was reduced from 45 mg to 40 mg.

4) The number of patients in your unit increased from 9 to 12.

5) You increase an IV flow rate from 6.5 mL/h to 8 mL/h.

6) The number of tacos in the breakroom decreased from 12 to 5.

7) You got a merit raise from $47.45/h to $49.05/h.

8) Your patient, who you encouraged to exercise and watch his diet, weighed 205 lb one month ago and now weighs 195 lb.

9) A dosage increased from 10 mg b.i.d to 20 mg b.i.d.

10) A patient weighed 78 kg on Monday and still weighs 78 kg on Thursday.

11) You had to adjust an IV drip from 32 gtt/min to 38 gtt/min.

12) You start a diet and reduce your caloric intake from 4500 kcal/day to 2500 kcal/day.

13) You can now do 25 pushups but a month ago you could only do 10.

14) You have a spouse and two kids on Monday. On Tuesday you have triplets. What is the percent change in total family members?

15) You own 7 cats and go to the shelter and adopt 2 more cats.

16) You ran a marathon in 6 hours in 2016. In 2019 you run the same marathon in 5 hours.

17) The distance you drive to work is 8.0 miles. On Monday you average 40 mph and it takes you 12 minutes. On Tuesday you average 80 mph and it takes you 6 minutes.

a) Calculate percent change in speed.

b) Calculate the percent change in time of commute.

c) Calculate the percent change in distance traveled.

18) Your patient's serum potassium level decreased from 4.1 mEq/L to 3.9 mEq/L.

19) One of your nine cats leaves you to live with the neighbor (better food, more petting).

20) You watched your diet and exercised, and your LDL decreased from 130 mg/dL to 120 mg/dL.

21) You increased a Pitocin drip from 2 milliunits/minute to 3 milliunits/minute.

22) A patient had his atorvastatin dosage lowered from 80 mg once daily to 40 mg once daily.

23) You notice the 99 Cent Store raised the price of dental floss from 99 cents to 99.9 cents.

24) You turned 30 today. What percent change have you aged in the last year?

25) The physician reduced a patient's daily dose from 10 mg to zero.

Chapter 21
Ratio Strength

1) How many mg of active ingredient are in 400 mL of a 1:10,000 solution?

2) How many mcg are in 100 mL of a 1:100,000 solution?

3) You have a 10 mL vial which is labeled 1:10,000 and are asked to draw up 0.5 mg of drug. How many mL would you draw?

4) How many grams of active ingredient are in 60 mL of a 1:200 solution?

5) How many grams of active ingredient are in 500 g of a 1:50 w/w preparation?

6) You have a 50 mL vial which is labeled 1:1000 and are asked to draw up 1.2 mg. How many mL would you draw?

7) You have a solution which is 1:1000 w/v. What is the percent strength?

8) What is the percent strength of a 1:100 w/v solution?

9) How many grams of active ingredient are in 100 mL of a 1:10,000 solution?

10) You have a 100 mL vial which is labeled 1:1000. How many mg are in 50 mL of the solution?

Unit 6: Miscellaneous Subjects

Chapter 22: Reconstitution Calculations
Corresponding Chapter and pages in DCFNS: None. New material for this book.
Importance: 7/10. These problems show up occasionally on tests. Once you reconstitute the drug according to instructions, all the calculations are preformed like any other dosage calculation.

Chapter 23: Conversions Between mg and mEq
Corresponding Chapter and pages in DCFNS: Chapter 12, pp. 53-56.
Importance: 2/10. As nurses you will probably never be required to convert between mg and mEq, but it is important to understand what milliequivalents are. Also, you have come this far in the book, why not spend another 20 minutes and learn how to do these problems?

Chapter 24: Dosage Calculations Puzzles
Corresponding Chapter and pages in DCFNS: None. New material for this book.
Importance: 0/10 You will never have problems like these on a nursing test or in real life, but you might find them amusing.

Chapter 25: Self-Assessment Exam
Corresponding Chapter and pages in DCFNS: Unit 4, pp. 57-61.
Importance: 10/10. It is important you test your knowledge. Check your answers and work on your weak areas, if any.

Chapter 22
Reconstitution Calculations

Some drugs come in a dry form and must be reconstituted before administration. The instructions for reconstitution will either be supplied with the drug or available in a data base and must be followed exactly.

The basic method of solving these problems:

- Reconstitute the drug according to the instructions.
- Look at the final concentration and volume when doing the calculations. Forget about the amount of diluent you added in the first step as this has nothing to do with the dosage calculations.
- Note: If you are given a nursing student test question which only gives the amount of diluent, with no information on the final volume or concentration, you do not have enough information to solve the problem. You can't assume that the diluent volume is equal to the final volume.

Example: A 500 mg vial has directions to reconstitute with 1.8 mL of diluent for a final concentration of 250 mg/mL. You have an order for 300 mg. How many mL will you withdraw to administer this dose?

$$300 \text{ mg} \left(\frac{1 \text{ mL}}{250 \text{ mg}}\right) = 1.2 \text{ mL}$$

Once you have reconstituted the vial, the amount of diluent is not a factor in the dosage calculation.

1) A 1 g vial states to add 8.1 mL of SW for injection for a final concentration of 100 mg/mL. You have an order for 250 mg IV. How many mL will you administer?

2) The physician has ordered 300 mg IM of a drug which is available in a 1000 mg vial with directions to add 4.6 mL SW for injection for a final concentration of 200 mg/mL. How many mL will you administer?

3) You have an order for 400 mg IM of a drug which is available in 1 g vials with directions to reconstitute with 8.5 mL of SW for injection for a final concentration of 100 mg/mL. How many mL will you administer?

4) A 1,000,000-unit vial of penicillin G potassium has instructions which state to reconstitute to a concentration of 100,000 units per mL, add 10 mL SW for injection. You have an order for 200,000 units IM. How many mL will you administer?

5) A 65 kg male patient diagnosed with herpes simplex encephalitis is to receive acyclovir 10 mg/kg IV infused over 1 hour, every 8 hours for 10 days. You have on hand a 1000 mg vial with the instructions to dissolve the contents of the vial in 20 mL of SWFI with the resulting solution containing 50 mg of acyclovir per mL. The calculated dose will then be withdrawn and added to a 100 mL bag of D5W. After reconstitution, what volume of the 50 mg/mL solution will you add to the 100 mL bag?

6) You are reconstituting a 150 mL bottle of amoxicillin 250 mg/5 mL. The instructions for reconstitution are as follows. Total amount of water required for reconstitution is 111 mL. Tap the bottle until all powder flows freely. Add approximately 1/3 of the total amount of water for reconstitution and shake vigorously to wet the powder. Add the remainder of the water and again shake vigorously. How long would the bottle last if the child were to take 5 mL PO t.i.d.?

7) A patient has an order for azithromycin 500 mg IV administered over 60 minutes at a concentration of 1 mg/mL. The 500 mg vial states: Prepare the initial solution of azithromycin for injection by adding 4.8 mL of Sterile Water For Injection to the vial and shaking the vial until all of the drug is dissolved. Each mL of the solution contains 100 mg of azithromycin.

a) The 5 mL vial will now be added to what size bag of NS to achieve a 1 mg/mL concentration?

b) At what rate will you set the IV infusion pump to the nearest tenth mL/h?

8) A patient has an order for streptomycin 500 mg IM which is available in 1 g vials with instructions to add 3.2 mL of Water for Injection USP for a final concentration of 250 mg/mL. How many mL will you administer?

9) You have an order for 250 mg IM of a drug which is available in a 500 mg vial with instructions to add 4.3 mL of SW for injection for a final concentration of 100 mg/mL. How many mL will you administer?

10) The physician has ordered 200 mg IM of a drug which is available in 1 g vials with instructions to add 3.5 mL SW for injection for a final concentration of 250 mg/mL. How many mL will you administer?

Chapter 23
Conversions Between mg and mEq

1) How many g of sodium acetate are in 16 mEq of sodium acetate?

2) How many grams of Na⁺ (just the sodium) are contained in 2.5 L of 10% NaCl?

3) How many mEq of NaCl are in 3 L of 0.9% NaCl?

4) How many mEq of calcium chloride are contained in 1.5 g of calcium chloride?

5) How many mEq of Ca⁺⁺ are in 2.4 g of calcium chloride?

6) How many mEq of K⁺ are contained in 240 mg of KCl?

7) How many mg of magnesium sulfate are in 20 mEq of magnesium sulfate?

8) How many mEq of KCl are in 15 mL of 10% KCl solution?

9) How many mEq of MgSO₄ are contained in 14 g of MgSO₄?

10) How many mg of KCl are in 30 mL of 2 mEq/mL KCl?

Chapter 24
Dosage Calculations Puzzles

These problems are just for fun and would never happen in a clinical setting. Also, they don't count as part of the 777 questions, so you are still getting your money's worth if you don't do them.

1) You have an order for 1 g of a drug to infuse over 2 hours. The pharmacy sends you a 1 L bag with a note saying: This bag contains 250 mL of 2 mg/mL, 250 mL of 1 mg/mL, 250 mL of 5 mg/mL and 250 mL of NS.

a) At what rate will you set the pump?

b) You started the infusion at 1300. You check on the patient at 1400 only to learn that the patient turned off the pump at 1330 because his friend told him that he didn't need any big pharma drugs. After explaining the importance of the drug to the patient, you get out your calculator and note pad. At what rate will you set the pump to finish the 1 g infusion on time if you restart the infusion at 1345?

2) You have an order to start an IV infusion at x mL/h, where $6x + 40 = 100$, on your patient Mr. Smith. The IV bag contains y mg/ z mL, where $2y + z = 1500$ and $z - y = 750$. Mr. Smith weighs 83 kg. How many mcg/kg/min is Mr. Smith receiving?

3) A new miracle drug is released by the FDA which reverses aging by 25% in adults over 50 YO. The dosage is 2 mg/kg + 1.5 mg for each year over 50 years old, rounded to the nearest 10 mg, given IV over 2 hours. The drug is available in 10 mg vials with instructions to reconstitute each vial with 8 mL of supplied diluent to yield a concentration of 1 mg/mL. Your facility's protocol is to reconstitute the appropriate number of vials and add to a 500 mL bag of D5W after withdrawing an equal volume of reconstituted drug from the 500 mL bag, then infuse over 2 hours. The drug, Gobakntime, is very expensive at $200/mg. Your facility has a new policy stating that the nurse who administers the drug must also calculate the charge of the drug and collect the cash payment. Your patient, Auld Guy, is 64 years old and weighs 82 kg. He is a little concerned about the price of the drug and relays to you that he makes $23.50/hour as a professional dog food taster. Auld Guy works 8 hours/day, five days per week. What will be the total charge for Auld Guy's therapy and how many weeks, days and hours will he have to work to pay for it?

Chapter 25
Self-Assessment Exam

The exam has 100 questions, each worth one point.

Convert the following:

1) 50 mL = ____ L

2) 6.5 g = ____ mg

3) 3 tbs = ____ mL

4) 1 cup = ____ mL

5) 90 mL = ____ fl oz

6) 182 lb = ____ kg

7) 6.5 cm = ____ in

8) 0.85 kg = ____ lb

9) 150 g = ____ kg

10) 3 tbs = ____ mL

Round the following numbers to the nearest tenth.

11) 6.45

12) 0.175

13) 8.97

14) 0.0002

15) 98.045

Round the following numbers to the nearest hundredth.

16) 6.875

17) 4.058

18) 30.005

19) 0.0555

20) 2.178

Write the corresponding Roman numerals for the following numbers:

21) 4

22) 9

23) 20

24) 53

25) 120

Write the corresponding numbers for the following Roman numerals:

26) VII

27) XIX

28) XXX

29) CIX

30) CCX

Convert the following to scientific notation:

31) 780,000

32) 142,000,000

33) 0.00054

34) 450

35) 549,000

Convert the following from scientific notation to numbers.

36) 5.34×10^4

37) 9.352×10^6

38) 1.502×10^{-5}

39) 5.1×10^{-6}

40) 2.004×10^7

Answer the following questions concerning military time.

41) You started studying for your exam at 1900 and finished at 2230. How many hours and minutes did you study?

42) What is 3:25 PM in military time?

43) You start and IV at 1000 which is scheduled to run 8 hours. What time will it end in military time?

44) A patient is to receive a medication every 8 hours around the clock. He received doses at 0600 and 1400. When should he receive the next dose?

45) You are asked to work from 11:00 AM to 1800. Your employer tells you that you can either be paid $35.00 per hour or a flat rate of $265. Which is the better deal for you?

Convert the following numbers to percents.

46) 0.05

47) 1.25

48) 0.45

Convert the following percents to numbers.

49) 23.1%

50) 100%

51) 0.15%

Express the following as percent strength solutions and include the type of solution (w/w, w/v, v/v, v/w).

52) 9 g NaCl in 1000 mL

53) 1 g KCl in 10 mL

54) 40 mL ETOH in 160 mL.

Answer the following:

55) How many mg of lidocaine are in 200 mL of 1% lidocaine solution?

56) How many mg of triamcinolone are in 30 g of 0.5% triamcinolone cream?

57) How many mg of NaCl are in 500 mL of 0.9% NaCl?

Answer the following questions pertaining to percent change.

58) You weigh 160 lb on August 1st and spend the next week hiking around Yosemite National Park. On August 8th you weigh 152 lb. What is the percent change in your weight?

59) You have two hamsters who fall in love and have 3 babies. What is the percent change in your hamster population?

60) The physician changed a patient's dose of a drug from 50 mg to 25 mg. What is the percent change in the dose?

61) Kristina F, a nursing student, scored 80% on her dosage calculation quiz on Monday. The following Monday she scored 90%. What is the percent change in her grade?

62) Your patient weighed 75 kg on admission and now weighs 72 kg. What is the percent change in the patient's weight?

Answer the following dosage questions.

63) The PCP has ordered 100 mg IM of a drug which is available in 200 mg/mL. How many mL will you administer?

64) The physician has ordered 30 mg IV of a drug which is available in 5 mL vials of 10 mg/mL. How many mL will you administer?

65) The NP ordered 50 mg PO once daily for a patient. The drug is available in 25 mg tablets. How many tablets will the patient take each day?

66) The physician has ordered 90 mg IM of a drug which is available in 5 mL vials containing 45 mg/mL. How many mL will you administer?

67) Your patient has an order for 12.5 mg PO of a drug which is available in 5 mg scored tablets. How many tabs will you administer?

68) Your 52 YO patient, who weighs 165 lb, has an order for drug xyz 100 mg/day divided into two doses. Drug xyz is available in 10 mL vials containing 50 mg/mL. How many mL will you administer per dose?

69) You have an order to administer 100 mcg/day PO divided into two doses. You have 0.025 mg tablets available. How many tablets will you administer per dose?

70) Your patient has an order for 250 mg IV every 6 hours of a drug which is available in 10 mL vials containing 25 mg/mL. How many mL will be administered in 24 hours?

71) The physician has ordered 250 mcg IM of a drug which is available in 2 mL vials containing 0.5 mg/mL. How many mL will you administer?

72) The physician has ordered 40 mg IV of a drug which is available in 5 mL vials containing 20 mg/mL. How many mL will you administer?

73) A 45 lb child has an order for furosemide 2 mg/kg PO once daily. Furosemide oral solution is available in 60 mL bottles containing 10 mg/mL. How many mL will you administer per dose?

74) An 81 kg patient is to receive an initial bolus dose of a drug 0.085 mg/kg over at least 2 minutes. The drug is available in 4 mL vials containing 2.5 mg/mL. How many mL will you administer?

75) A 135 lb patient is to receive a single IV dose of ondansetron 0.15 mg/kg for prevention of nausea and vomiting. Ondansetron is available in 20 mL MDV of 2 mg/mL. How many mL will you administer?

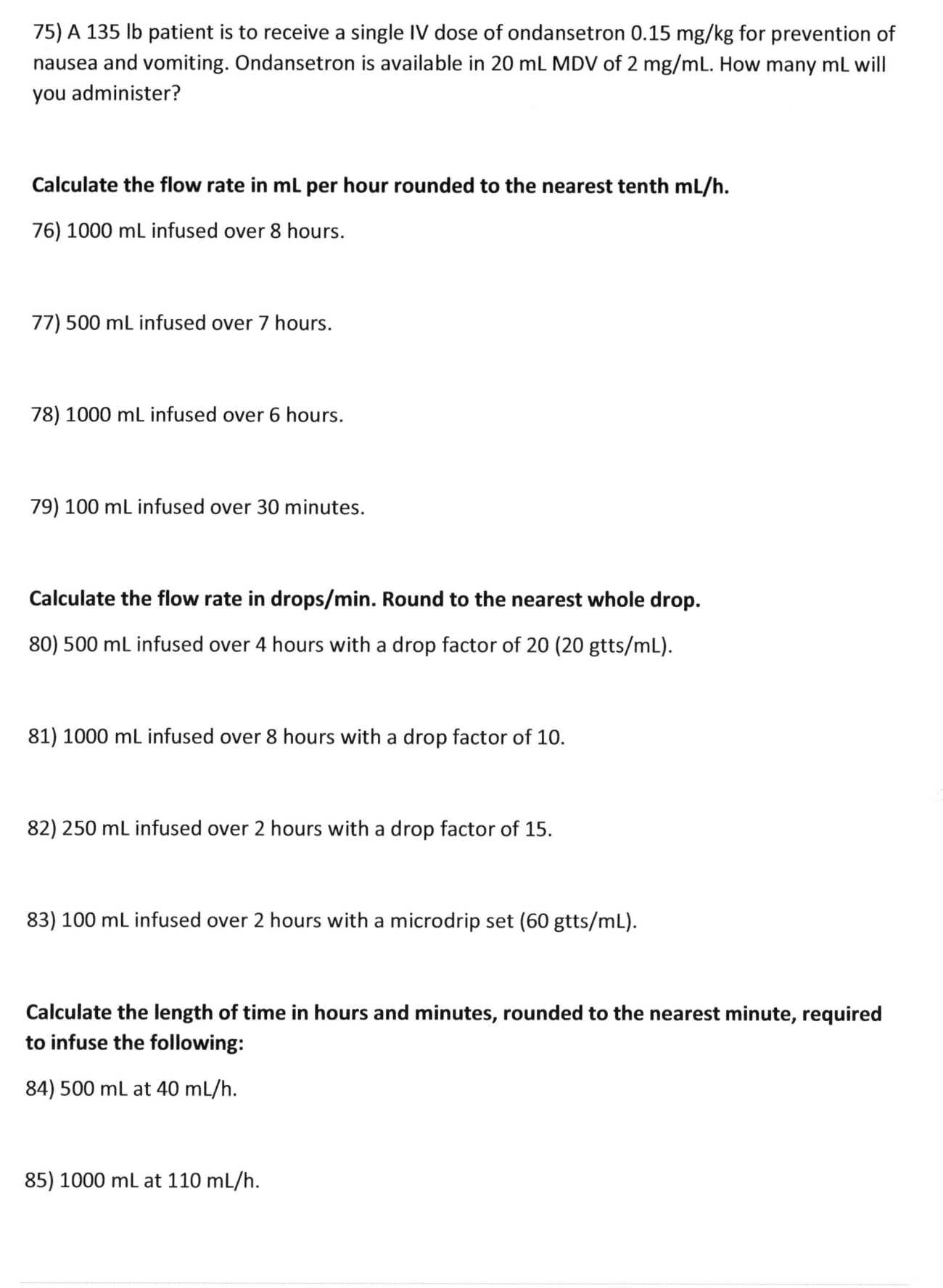

Calculate the flow rate in mL per hour rounded to the nearest tenth mL/h.

76) 1000 mL infused over 8 hours.

77) 500 mL infused over 7 hours.

78) 1000 mL infused over 6 hours.

79) 100 mL infused over 30 minutes.

Calculate the flow rate in drops/min. Round to the nearest whole drop.

80) 500 mL infused over 4 hours with a drop factor of 20 (20 gtts/mL).

81) 1000 mL infused over 8 hours with a drop factor of 10.

82) 250 mL infused over 2 hours with a drop factor of 15.

83) 100 mL infused over 2 hours with a microdrip set (60 gtts/mL).

Calculate the length of time in hours and minutes, rounded to the nearest minute, required to infuse the following:

84) 500 mL at 40 mL/h.

85) 1000 mL at 110 mL/h.

86) 500 mL at 35 gtts/min with a drop factor of 20.

87) 1 L at 30 gtts/min with a drop factor of 15.

Calculate the volume infused in the following scenarios.

88) Infusion rate of 30 mL/h for 4 h 30 min.

89) Infusion rate of 28 gtts/min, drop factor 20, for 3 hours 15 min.

Calculate the following. Round all drops/min to the nearest drop and all mL/h rates to the nearest tenth mL/h.

90) Your 67 kg patient has an order for a lidocaine infusion at the rate of 30 mcg/kg/min. You have a 250 mL bag labeled "Lidocaine HCl and 5% Dextrose Injection USP". Lidocaine 2 g (8 mg/mL) is printed in big red letters in the middle of the label. What rate will you set the IV infusion pump?

91) Your 140 lb patient, who has been diagnosed with septic shock, has an order for norepinephrine 0.15 mcg/kg/min IV. The pharmacy delivers a bag containing 4 mg norepinephrine in 250 mL D5NS. At what rate will you set the IV infusion pump?

92) Your 140 lb female patient has an order for dobutamine 5 mcg/kg/min IV to start at 1100. The dobutamine is available as 1000 mcg/mL. At what rate will you set the IV infusion pump?

Answer the following reconstitution calculation questions.

93) You have an order for 300 mg IM of a drug which is available in 1 g vials with directions to reconstitute with 7.5 mL of SW for injection for a final concentration of 100 mg/mL. How many mL will you administer?

94) A patient has an order for 500 mg IM of a drug which is available in 1 g vials with instructions to add 3.1 mL of Water for Injection USP for a final concentration of 250 mg/mL. How many mL will you administer?

Calculate the BSA in m² for the following people using the Mosteller formula.

95) An adult male weighing 185 lb and 5 ft 10 in tall.

96) A 14-month-old girl weighing 23 lb and 31 in tall.

97) An adult male weighing 214 lb and 6 ft 2 in tall.

Answer the following:

98) A mEq of Na⁺ and a mEq of K⁺ weigh the same. T or F

99) A mEq of Na⁺ and a mEq of K⁺ contain the same number of ions. T or F

100) Congratulations on finishing the self-assessment exam. It is important to be confident in your dosage calculations. T or F.

A Final Note

It is our hope that you found this book valuable and worthy of your study time. If so, please leave a review at www.nursesuperhero.com/dcw-review. If not, please let us know how we can improve the book by contacting us at support@nursesuperhero.com.

Chase Hassen and Brad Wojcik

List of Abbreviations and Symbols

Term	Meaning	Term	Meaning
%	percent	mcg	microgram
AI	active ingredient	MD	Doctor of Medicine
AOM	acute otitis media	MDV	multiple dose vial
b.i.d.	twice daily	mg	milligram
BEACOPP	a chemotherapy regimen	mL	milliliter
BSA	body surface area	mm	millimeter
cap	capsule	NP	Nurse Practitioner
cm	centimeter	NPO	nothing orally
D5NS	5% dextrose in normal saline	NS	normal saline
D5W	5% dextrose in water	NTG	nitroglycerin
DCFMS	*Dosage Calculations for Nursing Students*	OM	otitis media
dL	deciliter	oz	ounce
DVT	deep vein thrombosis	p.	page
ETOH	ethyl alcohol	PA	Physician Assistant
fl oz	fluid ounce	PCI	percutaneous coronary intervention
g	gram	PE	pulmonary embolism
gal	gallon	PO	orally
gr	grain	pp.	pages
gtt	drop	pt	pint or patient
gtts	drops	q	every
G-tube	gastrostomy tube	q 2 h	every 2 hours
h	hour	q 6 h	every 6 hours
HC	hydrocortisone	q.i.d.	four times daily
HSE	herpes simplex encephalitis	STEMI	ST-Elevation Myocardial Infarction
IM	Intramuscularly	SW	sterile water
in	inch	SWFI	sterile water for injection
INR	international normalized ratio	t.i.d.	three times daily
IV	intravenously	tab	tablet
IVP	IV push	tbs	tablespoonful
kg	kilogram	tsp	teaspoonful
L	liter	VZV	varicella zoster virus
lb	pound	Xa	activated Factor X (ten)
LDL	low-density lipoprotein	YO	years old
m	meter		

Answers to Exercises
Chapter 1
Rounding Numbers (Include trailing zeros.)

	Round to the Nearest Tenth	Rounded Number		Round to the Nearest Hundredth	Rounded Number
1	6.47	**6.5**	26	89.568	**89.57**
2	3.15	**3.2**	27	45.789	**45.79**
3	0.06	**0.1**	28	1.005	**1.01**
4	23.49	**23.5**	29	2.895	**2.90**
5	6.999	**7.0**	30	3.997	**4.00**
6	1.447	**1.4**	31	7.894	**7.89**
7	16.24	**16.2**	32	3.433	**3.43**
8	149.10	**149.1**	33	2.222	**2.22**
9	10.011	**10.0**	34	1.111	**1.11**
10	9.97	**10.0**	35	8.895	**8.90**
11	1001.89	**1001.9**	36	29.999	**30.00**
12	21.46	**21.5**	37	56.451	**56.45**
13	0.059	**0.1**	38	3.4723	**3.47**
14	0.0010	**0.0**	39	6.7754	**6.78**
15	6.239	**6.2**	40	0.099	**0.10**
16	4.4499	**4.4**	41	5.773	**5.77**
17	5.97	**6.0**	42	9.065	**9.07**
18	6.37	**6.4**	43	7.436	**7.44**
19	78.467	**78.5**	44	61.7712	**61.77**
20	4.449	**4.4**	45	73.612	**73.61**
21	97.89	**97.9**	46	9.713	**9.71**
22	1.01	**1.0**	47	4.59	**4.59**
23	5.67	**5.7**	48	66.7812	**66.78**
24	23.2323	**23.2**	49	0.795	**0.80**
25	64.0	**64.0**	50	3.912	**3.91**

Chapter 2
Roman Numerals

Fill in the blanks with the corresponding Roman numeral.

Problem	Number	Roman Numeral	Prob #	Number	Roman Numeral
1	6	VI	11	8	VIII
2	9	IX	12	200	CC
3	50	L	13	178	CLXXVIII
4	2	II	14	99	XCIX
5	49	XLIX	15	30	XXX
6	9	IX	16	35	XXXV
7	22	XXII	17	½	SS
8	100	C	18	4	IV
9	20	XX	19	2004	MMIV
10	33	XXXIII	20	36	XXXVI

Fill in the blanks with the corresponding number.

Problem	Roman Numeral	Number	Prob #	Roman Numeral	Number
21	V	5	31	XLIV	44
22	IV	4	32	DL	550
23	XX	20	33	CDL	450
24	XC	90	34	III	3
25	CXI	111	35	VIII	8
26	XXXIV	34	36	LXVI	66
27	MCM	1900	37	CC	200
28	SS	½	38	CXC	190
29	XLI	41	39	MMXIX	2019
30	CI	101	40	XL	40

Chapter 3
Scientific Notation

Convert the following numbers to scientific notation.

Problem	Number	Coefficient	# of Places from New Decimal Point to end of Original Number	Coefficient X 10 Raised to the Number of Places the Decimal Point was Moved
Example	47,000	4.7	4	4.7×10^4
1	64,500	6.45	4	6.45×10^4
2	23,000,000	2.3	7	2.3×10^7
3	14,000	1.4	4	1.4×10^4
4	237,400,000	2.374	8	2.374×10^8
5	1,000,100	1.0001	6	1.0001×10^6
6	175,000	1.75	5	1.75×10^5
7	63,500,000	6.35	7	6.35×10^7
8	6,023,000,000	6.023	9	6.023×10^9
9	700,000	7	5	7×10^5
10	45,020,000	4.502	7	4.502×10^7

Convert the following decimal numbers to scientific notation.

Problem	Decimal Number	Coefficient	# of Places from New Decimal Point to Original Decimal Point	Coefficient X 10 Raised to the Negative Number of Places the Decimal Point was Moved
Example	0.031	3.1	2	3.1×10^{-2}
11	0.000167	1.67	4	1.67×10^{-4}
12	0.000061	6.1	5	6.1×10^{-5}
13	0.0004068	4.068	4	4.068×10^{-4}
14	0.0001975	1.975	4	1.975×10^{-4}
15	0.0002001	2.001	4	2.001×10^{-4}
16	0.000045	4.5	5	4.5×10^{-5}
17	0.00000052	5.2	7	5.2×10^{-7}
18	0.000068	6.8	5	6.8×10^{-5}
19	0.001983	1.983	3	1.983×10^{-3}
20	0.0024	2.4	3	2.4×10^{-3}

Convert the following numbers from scientific notation to numbers.

Problem	Scientific Notation	Coefficient	Exponent	# of Places to Move the Decimal Point to the Right	Number
Example	1.42×10^7	1.42	7	7	14,200,000
21	3.8×10^4	3.8	4	4	38,000
22	4×10^5	4	5	5	400,000
23	3.01×10^6	3.01	6	6	3,010,000
24	3.05×10^4	3.05	4	4	30,500
25	2.79×10^8	2.79	8	8	279,000,000
26	8.99×10^5	8.99	5	5	899,000
27	3.78×10^8	3.78	8	8	378,000,000
28	2.0×10^8	2.0	8	8	200,000,000
29	8.56×10^5	8.56	5	5	856,000
30	2.31×10^7	2.31	7	7	23,100,000

Convert the following decimal numbers from scientific notation to decimal numbers.

Problem	Scientific Notation	Coefficient	Exponent	# of Places to Move the Decimal Point to the Left	Decimal Number
Example	3.04×10^{-4}	3.04	-4	4	0.000304
31	9.4×10^{-6}	9.4	-6	6	0.0000094
32	2.81×10^{-5}	2.81	-5	5	0.0000281
33	3.5×10^{-6}	3.5	-6	6	0.0000035
34	6.95×10^{-8}	6.95	-8	8	0.0000000695
35	3.3×10^{-9}	3.3	-9	9	0.0000000033
36	9.00×10^{-4}	9.00	-4	4	0.000900
37	1.42×10^{-3}	1.42	-3	3	0.00142
38	2.02×10^{-3}	2.02	-3	3	0.00202
39	9.6×10^{-7}	9.6	-7	7	0.00000096
40	5.4×10^{-5}	5.4	-5	5	0.000054

Chapter 4
Military Time

Convert the following civilian times to military time.

1) 3:25 AM   **0325**

2) 11:35 AM   **1135**

3) 2:29 PM   **1429**

4) 10:20 PM   **2220**

5) 4:00 PM   **1600**

Convert the following military times to civilian times.

6) 0318   **3:18 AM**

7) 2309   **11:09 PM**

8) 1004   **10:04 AM**

9) 1615   **4:15 PM**

10) 1309   **1:09 PM**

11) An IV was started at 1000 and ended at 3:30 PM. How long did it run in hours and minutes?

5 hours 30 min

12) A patient was admitted at 0900 on Tuesday and was discharged at 2:30 PM on the following day. How many hours did the patient spend in the hospital?

29.5 hours

13) A civilian time day has 24 hours. How many hours does a military time day have?

24 hours

14) You start work at 0700 at your hospital in California and take a lunch break at noon. You phone your friend in New York during lunch and after visiting for a while she looks at her watch and says, "It is 1530, I have to get back to work." What time is it in California?

1230

15) You have the day off and plan to run some errands. You leave the house at 0830, drive for 20 minutes to the coffee shop, spend 30 minutes enjoying your coffee, arrive at the grocery store at 9:45 AM, spend 30 minutes shopping, then arrive home 15 minutes after finishing shopping. What time is it in military time? **1030**

16) You have an order for 1 tablet PO q 8 h. You give the first dose at 0800. What time in military time will you give the next two doses?

1600 and 2400 (or 0000)

17) You start an IV at 1000 to run for 4 hours. What time in civilian time will it end?

2:00 PM

18) You have an order for 1 capsule q 6 h PO. You administer the first dose at 11:00 AM. What time in military time will you administer the third dose?

2300

19) Your cat is normally fed at 1700, but due to excessive meowing, you feed her at 4:30 PM. How many minutes early was she fed?

30 minutes

20) You start an IV at 2300 on Monday and it finishes at 0530 on Tuesday. How long did it run?

6 hours 30 minutes

Chapter 5
Unit Conversions Within the Metric System

Problem	Given to be Converted	Conversion Factor	Answer
Example	2.5 g	1000 mg/g =	2500 mg
1	1.3 g	1000 mg/g =	1300 mg
2	45 mL	1 L/1000 mL =	0.045 L
3	25 mL	1 dL/100 mL =	0.25 dL
4	65 mg	1 g/1000 mg =	0.065 g
5	4 cm	10 mm/cm =	40 mm
6	340 mcg	1 mg/1000 mcg =	0.34 mg
7	590 g	1 kg/1000 g =	0.59 kg
8	7.8 g	1000 mg/g =	7800 mg
9	2.1 L	1000 mL/L =	2100 mL
10	98 mm	1 cm/10 mm =	9.8 cm
11	6 mcg	1 mg/1000 mcg =	0.006 mg
12	800 mL	1 L/1000 mL =	0.8 L
13	5 mL	1 L/1000 mL =	0.005 L
14	87 mcg	1 mg/1000 mcg =	0.087 mg
15	650 mcg	1 mg/1000 mcg =	0.65 mg
16	6700 mcg	1 g/1,000,000 mcg =	0.0067 g
17	5 mg	1000 mcg/mg =	5000 mcg
18	78,000 mcg	1 g/1,000,000 mcg =	0.078 g
19	0.013 L	10 dL/L =	0.13 dL
20	2.2 kg	1000 g/kg =	2200 g
21	145 mcg	1 mg/1000 mcg =	0.145 mg
22	24 mL	1 L/1000 mL =	0.024 L
23	1.01 m	100 cm/m =	101 cm
24	250 mcg	1 mg/1000 mcg =	0.25 mg
25	3750 g	1 kg/1000 g =	3.75 kg
26	45 cm	1 m/100 cm =	0.45 m
27	4.1 L	1000 mL/L =	4100 mL
28	100 mL	1 L/1000 mL =	0.1 L
29	610 mL	1 dL/100 mL =	6.1 dL
30	1.05 L	1000 mL/L =	1050 mL

Chapter 6
Unit Conversions Within the Household System

Problem	Given to be Converted	Conversion Factor	Answer
Example	2 cups	8 fl oz/cup =	16 fl oz
1	2 fl oz	2 tbs/fl oz =	4 tbs
2	0.5 pt	16 fl oz/pt =	8 fl oz
3	2 gal	4 qt/gal =	8 qt
4	8 oz	1 lb/16 oz =	0.5 lb
5	12 fl oz	1 cup/8 fl oz =	1.5 cup
6	2 fl oz	6 tsp/fl oz =	12 tsp
7	6 tsp	1 tbs/3 tsp =	2 tbs
8	1 cup	8 fl oz/cup =	8 fl oz
9	4 fl oz	1 cup/8 fl oz =	0.5 cup
10	1 cup	1 pt/2 cups =	0.5 pt
11	2 pt	1 gal/8 pt =	0.25 gal
12	1 gal	8 pt/gal =	8 pt
13	4 tsp	1 fl oz/6 tsp =	0.67 fl oz
14	4 fl oz	2 tbs/fl oz =	8 tbs
15	2 tsp	1 tbs/3 tsp =	0.67 tbs
16	2 qt	4 cups/qt =	8 cups
17	2 cups	8 fl oz/cup =	16 fl oz
18	6 tsp	1 fl oz/6 tsp =	1 fl oz
19	4 pt	1 qt/2 pt =	2 qt
20	32 oz	1 lb/16 oz =	2 lb
21	1 pt	16 fl oz/pt =	16 fl oz
22	3 fl oz	2 tbs/fl oz =	6 tbs
23	6 fl oz	2 tbs/fl oz =	12 tbs
24	2 tbs	3 tsp/tbs =	6 tsp
25	3 cups	1 pt/2 cups =	1.5 pt
26	1 fl oz	6 tsp/fl oz =	6 tsp
27	8 fl oz	1 pt/16 fl oz =	0.5 pt
28	0.5 qt	32 fl oz/qt =	16 fl oz
29	1 gal	128 fl oz/gal =	128 fl oz
30	4 cups	1 pt/2 cups =	2 pt

Chapter 7
Unit Conversions Between Metric, Household and Apothecary Systems

Note: Use 1 gr = 60 mg for these conversions. This differs from DCFNS, which uses 1 gr = 65 mg.

Problem	Given to be Converted	Conversion Factor	Answer
Example	5 in	2.54 cm/in =	12.7 cm
1	2 gr	60 mg/gr =	120 mg
2	45 lb	1 kg/2.2 lb =	20.5 kg
3	1.5 cup	240 mL/cup =	360 mL
4	60 mL	1 fl oz/30 mL =	2 fl oz
5	7 in	2.54 cm/in =	17.8 cm
6	200 g	1 lb/454 g =	0.44 lb
7	3 tsp	5 mL/tsp =	15 mL
8	90 mL	1 cup/240 mL =	0.38 cup
9	3.5 fl oz	30 mL/fl oz =	105 mL
10	98 mm	1 in/25.4 mm =	3.9 in
11	3 gr	60 mg/gr =	180 mg
12	2 tsp	5 mL/tsp =	10 mL
13	1.5 fl oz	30 mL/fl oz =	45 mL
14	4 gr	60 mg/gr =	240 mg
15	18 in	2.54 cm/in =	45.7 cm
16	3 fl oz	30 mL/fl oz =	90 mL
17	2 tbs	15 mL/tbs =	30 mL
18	0.5 pt	480 mL/pt =	240 mL
19	2.2 kg	2.2 lb/kg =	4.84 lb
20	120 mg	1 gr/60 mg =	2 gr
21	90 mL	1 fl oz/30 mL =	3 fl oz
22	180 mg	1 gr/60 mg =	3 gr
23	4 fl oz	30 mL/fl oz =	120 mL
24	700 g	1 lb/454 g =	1.54 lb
25	180 mL	1 fl oz/30 mL =	6 fl oz
26	2 cups	8 fl oz/cup =	16 fl oz
27	454 g	1 lb/454 g=	1 lb
28	5 gr	60 mg/gr =	300 mg

Chapter 8
Dosage Calculations Level 1

Problem	Order	Available	Administer
Example	50 mg	25 mg/mL	50 mg (1 mL/25mg) = 2 mL
1	150 mg	50 mg/mL	150 mg (1 mL/50 mg) = 3 mL
2	500 mg	250 mg capsules	500 mg (1 cap/250 mg) = 2 caps
3	50 mcg	100 mcg/mL	50 mcg (1 mL/100 mcg) = 0.5 mL
4	0.5 g	0.25 g tab	0.5 g (1 tab/0.25 g) = 2 tabs
5	10 mg	20 mg/5 mL	10 mg (5 mL/20 mg) = 2.5 mL
6	0.25 mg	0.125 mg tabs	0.25 mg (1 tab/0.125 mg) = 2 tabs
7	600 mg	300 mg/2 mL	600 mg (2 mL/300 mg) = 4 mL
8	7.5 mg	5 mg scored tabs	7.5 mg (1 tab/5 mg) = 1.5 tabs
9	30 mg	15 mg/mL	30 mg (1 mL/15 mg) = 2 mL
10	0.125 mg	0.25 mg/mL	0.125 mg (1 mL/0.25 mg) = 0.5 mL
11	75 mg	50 mg/mL	75 mg (1 mL/50 mg) = 1.5 mL
12	1 g	0.25 g tab	1 g (1 tab/0.25 g) = 4 tabs
13	50 mcg	200 mcg/mL	50 mcg (1 mL/200 mcg) = 0.25 mL
14	1000 mg	500 mg tabs	1000 mg (1 tab/500 mg) = 2 tabs
15	1 mg	10 mg/mL	1 mg (1 mL/10 mg) = 0.1 mL
16	90 mg	60 mg/mL	90 mg (1 mL/60 mg) = 1.5 mL
17	250 mg	100 mg/mL	250 mg (1 mL/100 mg) = 2.5 mL
18	45 mg	50 mg/mL	45 mg (1 mL/50 mg) = 0.9 mL
19	0.25 g	0.5 g scored tabs	0.25 g (1 tab/0.5 g) = 0.5 tab
20	6 mg	3 mg/2 mL	6 mg (2 mL/3 mg) = 4 mL
21	100 mcg	25 mcg/mL	100 mcg (1 mL/25 mcg) = 4 mL
22	90 mg	200 mg/mL	90 mg (1 mL/200 mg) = 0.45 mL
23	8.5 mg	2 mg/mL	8.5 mg (1 mL/2 mg) = 4.3 mL
24	1 mg	0.5 mg/mL	1 mg (1 mL/0.5 mg) = 2 mL
25	15 mg	5 mg/5 mL	15 mg (5 mL/5 mg) = 15 mL
26	90 mg	20 mg/mL	90 mg (1 mL/20 mg) = 4.5 mL
27	0.6 mg	0.3 mg tabs	0.6 mg (1 tab/0.3 mg) = 2 tab

Problem	Order	Available	Administer
28	200 mcg	100 mcg/tab	200 mcg (1 tab/100 mcg) = 2 tabs
29	50 mg	100 mg/mL	50 mg (1 mL/100 mg) = 0.5 mL
30	150 mcg	50 mcg/mL	150 mcg (1 mL/50 mcg) = 3 mL
31	25 mg	12.5 mg/5 mL	25 mg (5 mL/12.5 mg) = 10 mL
32	3 mg	6 mg scored tab	3 mg (1 tab/6 mg) = 0.5 tab
33	20 mg	5 mg/mL	20 mg (1 mL/5 mg) = 4 mL
34	250 mcg	125 mcg tabs	250 mcg (1 tab/125 mcg) = 2 tabs
35	75 mg	150 mg/mL	75 mg (1 mL/150 mg) = 0.5 mL
36	3 mcg	1 mcg/mL	3 mcg (1 mL/1 mcg) = 3 mL
37	30 mg	10 mg/5 mL	30 mg (5 mL/10 mg) = 15 mL
38	5 mg	10 mg scored tab	5 mg (1 tab/10 mg) = 0.5 tab
39	7.5 mg	5 mg/mL	7.5 mg (1 mL/5 mg) = 1.5 mL
40	0.3 mg	0.1 mg tab	0.3 mg (1 tab/0.1 mg) = 3 tabs
41	250 mg	100 mg/mL	250 mg (1 mL/100 mg) = 2.5 mL
42	3.5 mg	1 mg/mL	3.5 mg (1 mL/1 mg) = 3.5 mL
43	480 mg	400 mg/5 mL	480 mg (5 mL/400 mg) = 6 mL
44	30 mg	150 mg/10 mL	30 mg (10 mL/150 mg) = 2 mL
45	500 mg	250 mg capsule	500 mg (1 cap/250 mg) = 2 caps
46	75 mg	25 mg/mL	75 mg (1 mL/25 mg) = 3 mL
47	1000 mg	500 mg/2 mL	1000 mg (2 mL/500 mg) = 4 mL
Problem	Order	Available	Adminster
48	20 mEq	10 mEq tab	20 mEq (1 tab/10 mEq) = 2 tabs
49	7.5 mg	5 mg/scored tab	7.5 mg (1 tab/5 mg) = 1.5 tabs
50	200 mg	100 mg capsule	200 mg (1 cap/100 mg) = 2 caps
51	5 mg	10 mg/mL	5 mg (1 mL/10 mg) = 0.5 mL
52	500 mg	250 mg/5 mL	500 mg (5 mL/250 mg) = 10 mL
53	20 mEq	20 mEq tab	20 mEq (1 tab/20 mEq) = 1 tab
54	2 mg	1 mg scored tab	2 mg (1 tab/1 mg) = 2 tabs
55	25 mg	50 mg scored tab	25 mg (1 mL/50 mg) = 0.5 tab
56	250 mg	125 mg/mL	250 mg (1 mL/125 mg) = 2 mL
57	7 mcg	10 mcg/10 mL	7 mcg (10 mL/10 mcg) = 7 mL
58	200 mg	100 mg capsule	200 mg (1 cap/100 mg) = 2 caps

Chapter 9
Dosage Calculations Level 2

1) The NP has ordered 100 mg IM b.i.d. of a drug which is available in 5 mL vials labeled 50 mg/mL. How many mL will you administer per dose?

$$\frac{100 \text{ mg}}{\text{dose}} \left(\frac{1 \text{ mL}}{50 \text{ mg}}\right) = \frac{2 \text{ mL}}{\text{dose}}$$

2) You have an order for 0.25 mg of levothyroxine which is available in 125 mcg scored tablets. How many tablets will you administer?

$$0.25 \text{ mg} \left(\frac{1 \text{ tab}}{125 \text{ mcg}}\right)\left(\frac{1000 \text{ mcg}}{\text{mg}}\right) = 2 \text{ tabs}$$

3) The physician has ordered drug xyz 50 mg/day IV divided into 2 doses. The pharmacy sends a 5 mL vial which contains drug xyz in a concentration of 100 mg/mL. How many mL will you administer for each dose?

$$\frac{50 \text{ mg}}{\text{day}} \left(\frac{1 \text{ day}}{2 \text{ doses}}\right)\left(\frac{1 \text{ mL}}{100 \text{ mg}}\right) = \frac{0.25 \text{ mL}}{\text{dose}}$$

4) Your 45 YO patient who weighs 178 lb has been ordered drug abc 100 mg/day IV divided into 4 doses. Drug abc is available in 10 mL vials containing 50 mg/mL. How many mL will you administer per dose?

$$\frac{100 \text{ mg}}{\text{day}} \left(\frac{1 \text{ day}}{4 \text{ doses}}\right)\left(\frac{1 \text{ mL}}{50 \text{ mg}}\right) = \frac{0.5 \text{ mL}}{\text{dose}}$$

5) The MD has ordered 100 mg PO t.i.d. of a drug which is available in 20 mL vials containing 50 mg/mL. How many mL will be administered each day?

$$\frac{100 \text{ mg}}{\text{dose}} \left(\frac{3 \text{ doses}}{\text{day}}\right)\left(\frac{1 \text{ mL}}{50 \text{ mg}}\right) = \frac{6 \text{ mL}}{\text{day}}$$

6) The provider has ordered 50 mcg/day PO divided into 2 doses. You have available 0.025 mg tablets. How many tablets will you administer per dose?

$$\frac{50 \text{ mcg}}{\text{day}} \left(\frac{1 \text{ day}}{2 \text{ dose}}\right)\left(\frac{1 \text{ tab}}{0.025 \text{ mg}}\right)\left(\frac{1 \text{ mg}}{1000 \text{ mcg}}\right) = \frac{1 \text{ tab}}{\text{dose}}$$

7) Your 67 YO patient has an order for 200 mg IM q 4 h. The drug is available as 100 mg/mL. How many mL will you administer per dose?

$$\frac{200 \text{ mg}}{\text{dose}} \left(\frac{1 \text{ mL}}{100 \text{ mg}}\right) = \frac{2 \text{ mL}}{\text{dose}}$$

8) The NP has ordered 1 g/day IV divided into 4 doses of a drug which is available in 20 mL vials containing 100 mg/mL. How many mL/dose will you administer?

$$\frac{1 \text{ g}}{\text{day}} \left(\frac{1 \text{ day}}{4 \text{ doses}}\right)\left(\frac{1 \text{ mL}}{100 \text{ mg}}\right)\left(\frac{1000 \text{ mg}}{\text{g}}\right) = \frac{2.5 \text{ mL}}{\text{dose}}$$

9) You have an order to administer a 400 mg dose IM of a drug which is available in 10 mL vials containing 1 g. How many mL will you administer?

$$400 \text{ mg} \left(\frac{10 \text{ mL}}{\text{g}}\right)\left(\frac{1 \text{ g}}{1000 \text{ mg}}\right) = 4 \text{ mL}$$

10) You have an order for 0.125 mg PO of a drug which is available in 125 mcg tablets. How many tablets do you administer?

$$0.125 \text{ mg} \left(\frac{1 \text{ tab}}{125 \text{ mcg}}\right)\left(\frac{1000 \text{ mcg}}{\text{mg}}\right) = 1 \text{ tab}$$

11) Your patient has been ordered 500 mg IV q 6 h of a drug which is available in 20 mL vials containing 25 mg/mL. How many mL will be administered in 24 hours?

$$\frac{500 \text{ mg}}{\text{dose}} \left(\frac{4 \text{ doses}}{\text{day}}\right)\left(\frac{1 \text{ mL}}{25 \text{ mg}}\right) = \frac{80 \text{ mL}}{\text{day}}$$

12) The order is for 1 g PO and you have 250 mg capsules available. How many capsules will you administer?

$$1 \text{ g} \left(\frac{1 \text{ cap}}{250 \text{ mg}}\right)\left(\frac{1000 \text{ mg}}{\text{g}}\right) = 4 \text{ caps}$$

13) You have an order for 500 mcg IV of drug xyz which is available in 5 mL vials labeled 0.25 mg/mL. How many mL will you administer?

$$500 \text{ mcg} \left(\frac{1 \text{ mL}}{0.25 \text{ mg}}\right)\left(\frac{1 \text{ mg}}{1000 \text{ mcg}}\right) = 2 \text{ mL}$$

14) The physician has ordered 1000 mg/day PO divided into 2 doses of a drug which is available in 250 mg capsules. How many capsules will you administer per dose?

$$\frac{1000 \text{ mg}}{\text{day}} \left(\frac{1 \text{ day}}{2 \text{ doses}}\right)\left(\frac{1 \text{ cap}}{250 \text{ mg}}\right) = \frac{2 \text{ caps}}{\text{dose}}$$

15) Your patient has an order for 1.5 mg IV of a drug which is available in 5 mL vials containing 500 mcg/mL. How many mL will you administer?

$$1.5 \text{ mg} \left(\frac{1 \text{ mL}}{500 \text{ mcg}}\right)\left(\frac{1000 \text{ mcg}}{1 \text{ mg}}\right) = 3 \text{ mL}$$

16) Your patient is to receive 12.5 mg PO q.i.d. You have 25 mg scored tablets available. How many tablets will the patient receive for each dose?

$$12.5 \text{ mg} \left(\frac{1 \text{ tab}}{25 \text{ mg}}\right) = 0.5 \text{ tab}$$

17) Your patient is to receive 120 mL of a commercial formula via G-Tube q.i.d. The formula is available in 240 mL containers. How many containers will be administered each day?

$$\frac{120 \text{ mL}}{\text{dose}} \left(\frac{4 \text{ doses}}{\text{day}}\right)\left(\frac{1 \text{ container}}{240 \text{ mL}}\right) = \frac{2 \text{ containers}}{\text{day}}$$

18) The healthcare provider has ordered 100 mg/day IV divided into 4 doses. You have a 5 mL vial labeled 50 mg/mL. How many mL will you administer per dose?

$$\frac{100 \text{ mg}}{\text{day}} \left(\frac{1 \text{ day}}{4 \text{ doses}}\right)\left(\frac{1 \text{ mL}}{50 \text{ mg}}\right) = \frac{0.5 \text{ mL}}{\text{dose}}$$

19) The order is for 0.5 g PO b.i.d. You have 250 mg capsules available. How many capsules will be administered per day?

$$\frac{0.5 \text{ g}}{\text{dose}} \left(\frac{2 \text{ doses}}{\text{day}}\right)\left(\frac{1 \text{ cap}}{250 \text{ mg}}\right)\left(\frac{1000 \text{ mg}}{\text{g}}\right) = \frac{4 \text{ caps}}{\text{day}}$$

20) Your patient has an order for 600 mg/day IV divided into 4 doses. You have available a 10 mL vial containing 500 mg of the drug. How many mL will you administer per dose?

$$\frac{600 \text{ mg}}{\text{day}} \left(\frac{1 \text{ day}}{4 \text{ doses}}\right) \left(\frac{10 \text{ mL}}{500 \text{ mg}}\right) = \frac{3 \text{ mL}}{\text{dose}}$$

21) The order is 500 mcg IV. On hand you have a 2 mL vial containing 1 mg/mL. How many mL will you administer?

$$500 \text{ mcg} \left(\frac{1 \text{ mL}}{\text{mg}}\right) \left(\frac{1 \text{ mg}}{1000 \text{ mcg}}\right) = 0.5 \text{ mL}$$

22) The PA has ordered 900 mcg IM of a drug which is available in 1 mL vials containing 2 mg/mL. How many mL will you administer?

$$900 \text{ mcg} \left(\frac{1 \text{ mL}}{2 \text{ mg}}\right) \left(\frac{1 \text{ mg}}{1000 \text{ mcg}}\right) = 0.45 \text{ mL}$$

23) The healthcare provider has ordered 4.5 mg IV t.i.d. for your patient. The drug is available in 10 mL vials containing 10 mg/mL. How many mL will you draw up to administer one dose?

$$4.5 \text{ mg} \left(\frac{1 \text{ mL}}{10 \text{ mg}}\right) = 0.45 \text{ mL}$$

24) The NP has ordered 3 mg IV for your 189 lb patient. The drug is available in 10 mL vials containing 500 mcg/mL. How many mL will you administer?

$$3 \text{ mg} \left(\frac{1 \text{ mL}}{500 \text{ mcg}}\right) \left(\frac{1000 \text{ mcg}}{\text{mg}}\right) = 6 \text{ mL}$$

25) Your patient has an order for 15 mg PO of a drug to be administer at 2100. You have available 7.5 mg capsules. How many capsules will you administer?

$$15 \text{ mg} \left(\frac{1 \text{ cap}}{7.5 \text{ mg}}\right) = 2 \text{ caps}$$

26) The physician has ordered 35 mg IV of a drug which is available in 5 mL vials containing 20 mg/mL. How many mL will you administer?

$$35 \text{ mg} \left(\frac{1 \text{ mL}}{20 \text{ mg}}\right) = 1.8 \text{ mL}$$

27) The physician has ordered 0.8 mg IV q 2 h for 2 doses. You have available 5 mL vials containing 0.4 mg/mL. How many mL will you administer for one dose?

$$0.8 \text{ mg} \left(\frac{1 \text{ mL}}{0.4 \text{ mg}}\right) = 2 \text{ mL}$$

28) Your pediatric patient will be going home with a 150 mL bottle of amoxicillin 250 mg/5 mL with instructions for 5 mL to be given PO q 8 h. How long will the bottle last?

$$150 \text{ mL} \left(\frac{1 \text{ dose}}{5 \text{ mL}}\right) \left(\frac{1 \text{ day}}{3 \text{ doses}}\right) = 10 \text{ days}$$

29) The physician has ordered 100 mg/day IM divided into 2 doses. You have a 1 mL vial labeled 50 mg/mL. How many mL will you administer per dose?

$$\frac{100 \text{ mg}}{\text{day}} \left(\frac{1 \text{ day}}{2 \text{ doses}}\right) \left(\frac{1 \text{ mL}}{50 \text{ mg}}\right) = \frac{1 \text{ mL}}{\text{dose}}$$

30) You have an order for 1 g/day PO divided into 2 doses. You have 250 mg tablets available. How many tablets will you administer per dose?

$$\frac{1\text{ g}}{\text{day}}\left(\frac{1\text{ day}}{2\text{ doses}}\right)\left(\frac{1\text{ tab}}{250\text{ mg}}\right)\left(\frac{1000\text{ mg}}{\text{g}}\right) = \frac{2\text{ tabs}}{\text{dose}}$$

Chapter 10
Dosage Calculations Level 3

1) A 74 kg patient is scheduled for a PCI and will receive an IV bolus dose of abciximab 0.25 mg/kg followed immediately by an infusion of the drug. The abciximab is available in 5 mL vials containing 2 mg/mL. How many mL will you administer for the bolus?

$$\frac{0.25 \text{ mg}}{\text{kg}} \left(\frac{74 \text{ kg}}{1}\right)\left(\frac{1 \text{ mL}}{2 \text{ mg}}\right) = 9.3 \text{ mL}$$

2) A 6 YO child weighing 50 lb is diagnosed with bacterial sinusitis and is prescribed azithromycin 10 mg/kg PO once daily for 3 days. Azithromycin oral suspension is available in 15 mL, 22.5 and 30 mL bottles containing 200 mg/5 mL. How many mL will you administer?

$$\frac{10 \text{ mg}}{\text{kg}} \left(\frac{50 \text{ lb}}{1}\right)\left(\frac{1 \text{ kg}}{2.2 \text{ lb}}\right)\left(\frac{5 \text{ mL}}{200 \text{ mg}}\right) = 5.7 \text{ mL}$$

3) A 172 lb patient with atrial fibrillation is to receive an initial IV bolus of verapamil 0.075 mg/kg over at least 2 minutes. The drug is available in 4 mL vials containing 2.5 mg/mL. How many mL will you administer?

$$\frac{0.075 \text{ mg}}{\text{kg}} \left(\frac{172 \text{ lb}}{1}\right)\left(\frac{1 \text{ kg}}{2.2 \text{ lb}}\right)\left(\frac{1 \text{ mL}}{2.5 \text{ mg}}\right) = 2.3 \text{ mL}$$

4) A 60 kg patient is to receive a single IV dose of ondansetron 0.15 mg/kg, in addition to other drugs, for prevention of chemotherapy-induced nausea and vomiting. Ondansetron is available in a MDV of 40 mg/ 20mL. How many mL will you administer?

$$\frac{0.15 \text{ mg}}{\text{kg}} \left(\frac{60 \text{ kg}}{1}\right)\left(\frac{20 \text{ mL}}{40 \text{ mg}}\right) = 4.5 \text{ mL}$$

5) A 6 YO 42 lb child with acute otitis media (AOM) is to receive oral amoxicillin 80 mg/kg/day divided every 12 hours. The amoxicillin is available in 75 mL bottles containing 400 mg/5 mL. How many mL will you administer per dose?

$$\frac{80 \text{ mg}}{\text{kg day}} \left(\frac{42 \text{ lb}}{1}\right)\left(\frac{1 \text{ kg}}{2.2 \text{ lb}}\right)\left(\frac{1 \text{ day}}{2 \text{ doses}}\right)\left(\frac{5 \text{ mL}}{400 \text{ mg}}\right) = \frac{9.5 \text{ mL}}{\text{dose}}$$

6) A 72 kg male diagnosed with bacterial meningitis has an order for gentamicin 5 mg/kg/day IV in divided doses every 8 hours. How many mg will you administer for each dose?

$$\frac{5 \text{ mg}}{\text{kg day}} \left(\frac{72 \text{ kg}}{1}\right)\left(\frac{1 \text{ day}}{3 \text{ doses}}\right) = \frac{120 \text{ mg}}{\text{dose}}$$

7) A 12-month-old 22 lb child has been prescribed a maintenance dose of digoxin 10 mcg/kg/day PO administered in equal divided doses twice daily. Digoxin elixir is available in 60 mL bottles containing 50 mcg/mL. How many mL will you administer per dose?

$$\frac{10 \text{ mcg}}{\text{kg day}} \left(\frac{22 \text{ lb}}{1}\right)\left(\frac{1 \text{ kg}}{2.2 \text{ lb}}\right)\left(\frac{1 \text{ day}}{2 \text{ doses}}\right)\left(\frac{1 \text{ mL}}{50 \text{ mcg}}\right) = \frac{1 \text{ mL}}{\text{dose}}$$

8) A 51 YO 145 lb patient diagnosed with meningitis has an order for amikacin 5 mg/kg IV every 8 hours for 14 days. The amikacin is available in 2 mL vials containing 500 mg. How many mL will you administer each dose?

$$\frac{5 \text{ mg}}{\text{kg dose}} \left(\frac{145 \text{ lb}}{1}\right)\left(\frac{1 \text{ kg}}{2.2 \text{ lb}}\right)\left(\frac{2 \text{ mL}}{500 \text{ mg}}\right) = \frac{1.3 \text{ mL}}{\text{dose}}$$

9) A 174 lb patient is to receive cephalexin 500 mg PO b.i.d. The drug is available in 250 mg capsules. How many capsules will the patient receive in a 24-hour period?

$$\frac{500 \text{ mg}}{\text{dose}} \left(\frac{2 \text{ doses}}{\text{day}}\right)\left(\frac{1 \text{ cap}}{250 \text{ mg}}\right) = \frac{4 \text{ caps}}{\text{day}}$$

10) A 45 YO 152 lb adult has an order for ceftazidime 90 mg/kg/day IV in divided doses every 8 hours. How many mg will you administer per dose?

$$\frac{90 \text{ mg}}{\text{kg day}} \left(\frac{152 \text{ lb}}{1}\right)\left(\frac{1 \text{ kg}}{2.2 \text{ lb}}\right)\left(\frac{1 \text{ day}}{3 \text{ doses}}\right) = \frac{2073 \text{ mg}}{\text{dose}}$$

11) A 4 YO 38 lb child with hypertension has be ordered furosemide 1 mg/kg/dose PO twice daily. Furosemide oral solution is available in 60 mL bottles containing 10 mg/mL. How many mL will you administer each dose?

$$\frac{1 \text{ mg}}{\text{kg dose}} \left(\frac{38 \text{ lb}}{1}\right)\left(\frac{1 \text{ kg}}{2.2 \text{ lb}}\right)\left(\frac{1 \text{ mL}}{10 \text{ mg}}\right) = \frac{1.7 \text{ mL}}{\text{dose}}$$

12) A 145 lb patient is to receive a single IV dose of ondansetron 0.15 mg/kg, in addition to other drugs, for prevention of chemotherapy-induced nausea and vomiting. Ondansetron is available in a 20 mL MDV of 2 mg/mL. How many mL will you administer?

$$\frac{0.15 \text{ mg}}{\text{kg}} \left(\frac{145 \text{ lb}}{1}\right)\left(\frac{1 \text{ kg}}{2.2 \text{ lb}}\right)\left(\frac{1 \text{ mL}}{2 \text{ mg}}\right) = 4.9 \text{ mL}$$

13) A 65 kg patient diagnosed with STEMI is to receive an IV bolus dose of abciximab 0.25 mg/kg followed by a maintenance infusion of the drug at the rate of 0.125 mcg/kg/min. The abciximab is available in 5 mL vials containing 2 mg/mL.

a) How many mL will you administer for the bolus?

$$\frac{0.25 \text{ mg}}{\text{kg}} \left(\frac{65 \text{ kg}}{1}\right)\left(\frac{1 \text{ mL}}{2 \text{ mg}}\right) = 8.1 \text{ mL}$$

b) How many mcg/min will the patient receive during the maintenance infusion?

$$\frac{0.125 \text{ mcg}}{\text{kg min}} \left(\frac{65 \text{ kg}}{1}\right) = \frac{8.1 \text{ mcg}}{\text{min}}$$

14) A 5 YO 38 lb child with a mild infection is to receive oral amoxicillin 40 mg/kg/day in divided doses every 8 hours. The amoxicillin is available in 150 mL bottles containing 250 mg/5 mL. How many mL will you administer per dose?

$$\frac{40 \text{ mg}}{\text{kg day}} \left(\frac{38 \text{ lb}}{1}\right)\left(\frac{1 \text{ kg}}{2.2 \text{ lb}}\right)\left(\frac{1 \text{ day}}{3 \text{ doses}}\right)\left(\frac{5 \text{ mL}}{250 \text{ mg}}\right) = \frac{4.6 \text{ mL}}{\text{dose}}$$

15) A 53 YO adult male weighing 168 lb, who is being treated for VZV encephalitis, has been prescribed acyclovir 10 mg/kg/dose IV q 8 h for 10 days. Acyclovir for injection is available in 10 and 20 mL vials containing 50 mg/mL.

a) How many mg will the patient receive each day?

$$\frac{10 \text{ mg}}{\text{kg dose}} \left(\frac{168 \text{ lb}}{1}\right)\left(\frac{1 \text{ kg}}{2.2 \text{ lb}}\right)\left(\frac{3 \text{ doses}}{\text{day}}\right) = \frac{2291 \text{ mg}}{\text{day}}$$

b) How many mg will be patient receive each dose?

$$\frac{10 \text{ mg}}{\text{kg dose}} \left(\frac{168 \text{ lb}}{1}\right)\left(\frac{1 \text{ kg}}{2.2 \text{ lb}}\right) = \frac{764 \text{ mg}}{\text{dose}}$$

c) How many mL will the patient receive each dose?

$$\frac{764 \text{ mg}}{\text{dose}} \left(\frac{1 \text{ mL}}{50 \text{ mg}}\right) = \frac{15.3 \text{ mL}}{\text{dose}}$$

d) How many mL will the patient receive each day?

$$\frac{15.3 \text{ mL}}{\text{dose}} \left(\frac{3 \text{ doses}}{\text{day}}\right) = \frac{45.9 \text{ mL}}{\text{day}}$$

16) A 158 lb adult male diagnosed with endocarditis has an order for gentamicin 3 mg/kg/day IV in 2 divided doses, in addition to vancomycin. The gentamicin is available in 2 mL vials containing 40 mg/mL. The facility protocol is to round the gentamicin dose to the nearest 10 mg, then calculate the volume of solution to the nearest tenth mL. How many mL will you administer per dose?

$$\frac{3 \text{ mg}}{\text{kg day}} \left(\frac{158 \text{ lb}}{1}\right)\left(\frac{1 \text{ kg}}{2.2 \text{ lb}}\right)\left(\frac{1 \text{ day}}{2 \text{ doses}}\right) = \frac{107.7 \text{ mg}}{\text{dose}} \text{ rounded to } \frac{110 \text{ mg}}{\text{dose}}$$

$$\frac{110 \text{ mg}}{\text{dose}} \left(\frac{1 \text{ mL}}{40 \text{ mg}}\right) = \frac{2.8 \text{ mL}}{\text{dose}}$$

17) A 7 YO 50 lb child has been prescribed a maintenance dose of digoxin 4 mcg/kg/day PO administered in equal divided doses twice daily. Digoxin elixir is available in 60 mL bottles containing 50 mcg/mL. How many mL will you administer per dose?

$$\frac{4 \text{ mcg}}{\text{kg day}} \left(\frac{50 \text{ lb}}{1}\right)\left(\frac{1 \text{ kg}}{2.2 \text{ lb}}\right)\left(\frac{1 \text{ day}}{2 \text{ doses}}\right)\left(\frac{1 \text{ mL}}{50 \text{ mcg}}\right) = \frac{0.9 \text{ mL}}{\text{dose}}$$

18) A 4 YO 35 lb child has an order for ceftazidime 40 mg/kg IV every 8 hours. How many mg will you administer per dose?

$$\frac{40 \text{ mg}}{\text{kg}} \left(\frac{35 \text{ lb}}{1}\right)\left(\frac{1 \text{ kg}}{2.2 \text{ lb}}\right) = 636 \text{ mg}$$

19) Drug xyz has the following dosing guidelines:

Initiate therapy at 8-10 mg/kg/day IV once daily for 2 days, then decrease dosage by 25% for days 3 and 4, then discontinue. The prescriber has ordered an initial dose of 9 mg/kg/day for a 59 YO 182 lb male. The drug is available in 10 mL vials labeled 100 mg/mL.

a) How many mL will you administer on day 1?

$$\frac{9 \text{ mg}}{\text{kg day}} \left(\frac{182 \text{ lb}}{1}\right)\left(\frac{1 \text{ kg}}{2.2 \text{ lb}}\right)\left(\frac{1 \text{ mL}}{100 \text{ mg}}\right) = \frac{7.4 \text{ mL}}{\text{day}} \text{ (on day 1)}$$

b) How many mL will you administer on day 3? (Assume patient's weight has not changed.)

9 mg (0.75)/kg/day = 6.75 mg/kg/day

$$\frac{6.75 \text{ mg}}{\text{kg day}} \left(\frac{182 \text{ lb}}{1}\right)\left(\frac{1 \text{ kg}}{2.2 \text{ lb}}\right)\left(\frac{1 \text{ mL}}{100 \text{ mg}}\right) = \frac{5.6 \text{ mL}}{\text{day}} \text{ (on day 3)}$$

20) A 3 YO 31 lb child with edema has be ordered furosemide 2 mg/kg PO once daily. Furosemide oral solution is available in 60 mL bottles containing 10 mg/mL. How many mL will you administer each day?

$$\frac{2 \text{ mg}}{\text{kg}} \left(\frac{31 \text{ lb}}{1}\right)\left(\frac{1 \text{ kg}}{2.2 \text{ lb}}\right)\left(\frac{1 \text{ mL}}{10 \text{ mg}}\right) = 2.8 \text{ mL}$$

21) A 7 YO child weighing 44 lb is diagnosed with bacterial sinusitis and is prescribed azithromycin 10 mg/kg PO once daily for 3 days. Azithromycin oral suspension is available in 15, 22.5 and 30 mL bottles containing 200 mg/5 mL. How many mL will you administer?

$$\frac{10 \text{ mg}}{\text{kg}} \left(\frac{44 \text{ lb}}{1}\right)\left(\frac{1 \text{ kg}}{2.2 \text{ lb}}\right)\left(\frac{5 \text{ mL}}{200 \text{ mg}}\right) = 5 \text{ mL}$$

22) Your 67 YO 195 lb, 5 ft 10 in male patient diagnosed with testicular cancer has been prescribed ifosfamide 1200 mg/m²/day for 5 days. You calculate the BSA using the Mosteller method as being 2.09 m². Ifosfamide is available in 60 mL vials containing 3 g of drug. How many mL will you administer each day?

$$\frac{1200 \text{ mg}}{\text{m}^2 \text{ day}} \left(\frac{2.09 \text{ m}^2}{1}\right)\left(\frac{60 \text{ mL}}{3 \text{ g}}\right)\left(\frac{1 \text{ g}}{1000 \text{ mg}}\right) = \frac{50.2 \text{ mL}}{\text{day}}$$

23) A 6 YO 44 lb child has been prescribed an initial loading dose of warfarin 0.2 mg/kg PO. Warfarin is available in 1 mg, 2 mg, 2.5 mg, 3 mg, 4 mg, 5 mg, 6 mg, 7.5 mg and 10 mg scored tablets.

a) How many mg will the child receive, and which tablet strength would you use?

$$\frac{0.2 \text{ mg}}{\text{kg}} \left(\frac{44 \text{ lb}}{1}\right)\left(\frac{1 \text{ kg}}{2.2 \text{ lb}}\right) = 4 \text{ mg}$$

The 4 mg tablet would be best, but you could also use 2 of the 2 mg tablets or 4 of the 1 mg tablets.

b) On day 2, the INR comes back at 3.2 with a dosing protocol to reduce dose to 25% of the initial loading dose. How many mg would you administer, and which tablet strength would you use?

$$4 \text{ mg } (0.25) = 1 \text{ mg} \quad \text{Use the 1 mg tablet.}$$

24) A 40 kg child has been prescribed an initial loading dose of warfarin 0.2 mg/kg PO. Warfarin is available in 1 mg, 2 mg, 2.5 mg, 3 mg, 4 mg, 5 mg, 6 mg, 7.5 mg and 10 mg scored tablets.

a) How many mg will the child receive, and which tablet strength would you use?

$$\frac{0.2 \text{ mg}}{\text{kg}} \left(\frac{40 \text{ kg}}{1}\right) = 8 \text{ mg Use 2 of the 4 mg tablets.}$$

b) On day 2, the INR comes back at 2.5 with a dosing protocol to reduce dose to 50% of the initial loading dose. How many mg would you administer, and which tablet strength would you use?

$$8 \text{ mg } (0.50) = 4 \text{ mg}$$

The 4 mg tablet would be best, but you could also use 2 of the 2 mg tablets or 4 of the 1 mg tablets.

25) A 42 YO adult male weighing 142 lb, who is being treated for HSE (herpes simplex encephalitis), has been prescribed acyclovir 10 mg/kg/dose IV q 8 h for 14 days. Acyclovir for injection is available in 10 and 20 mL vials containing 50 mg/mL.

a) How many mg will the patient receive each day?

$$\frac{10 \text{ mg}}{\text{kg dose}} \left(\frac{142 \text{ lb}}{1}\right)\left(\frac{1 \text{ kg}}{2.2 \text{ lb}}\right)\left(\frac{3 \text{ doses}}{\text{day}}\right) = \frac{1936 \text{ mg}}{\text{day}}$$

b) How many mg will be patient receive each dose?

$$\frac{10 \text{ mg}}{\text{kg dose}} \left(\frac{142 \text{ lb}}{1}\right)\left(\frac{1 \text{ kg}}{2.2 \text{ lb}}\right) = \frac{645 \text{ mg}}{\text{dose}}$$

c) How many mL will the patient receive each dose?

$$\frac{645 \text{ mg}}{\text{dose}} \left(\frac{1 \text{ mL}}{50 \text{ mg}}\right) = \frac{12.9 \text{ mL}}{\text{dose}}$$

d) How many mL will the patient receive each day?

$$\frac{12.9 \text{ mL}}{\text{dose}} \left(\frac{3 \text{ doses}}{\text{day}}\right) = \frac{38.7 \text{ mL}}{\text{day}}$$

26) Drug xyz has the following dosing guidelines:

Initiate therapy at 4 – 6 mg/kg/day IV once daily for 2 days, then decrease dosage by 25% for days 3 and 4, then discontinue. The prescriber has ordered an initial dose of 5 mg/kg/day for a 48 YO 176 lb male. The drug is available in 10 mL vials labeled 100 mg/mL.

a) How many mL will you administer on day 1?

$$\frac{5 \text{ mg}}{\text{kg day}} \left(\frac{176 \text{ lb}}{1}\right)\left(\frac{1 \text{ kg}}{2.2 \text{ lb}}\right)\left(\frac{1 \text{ mL}}{100 \text{ mg}}\right) = \frac{4 \text{ mL}}{\text{day}} \text{ (on day 1)}$$

b) How many mL will you administer on day 3? (Assume patient's weight has not changed.)

5 mg (0.75)/kg/day = 3.75 mg/kg/day

$$\frac{3.75 \text{ mg}}{\text{kg day}} \left(\frac{176 \text{ lb}}{1}\right)\left(\frac{1 \text{ kg}}{2.2 \text{ lb}}\right)\left(\frac{1 \text{ mL}}{100 \text{ mg}}\right) = \frac{3 \text{ mL}}{\text{day}} \text{ (on day 3)}$$

Or

$$\frac{4 \text{ mL}}{\text{day}} \left(\frac{0.75}{1}\right) = \frac{3 \text{ mL}}{\text{day}} \text{ (on day 3)}$$

27) A 160 lb patient diagnosed with supraventricular tachycardia is to receive verapamil 5 mg IV over 2 minutes. The drug is available in 4 mL vials containing 2.5 mg/mL. How many mL will you administer?

$$5 \text{ mg} \left(\frac{1 \text{ mL}}{2.5 \text{ mg}}\right) = 2 \text{ mL}$$

28) A 72 YO 183 lb patient diagnosed with an M. chelonae infection has an order for amikacin 15 mg/kg IV once daily for 2 weeks (in addition to a high dose of cefoxitin). The amikacin is available in 2 mL vials containing 500 mg. How many mL will you administer each day?

$$\frac{15 \text{ mg}}{\text{kg}} \left(\frac{183 \text{ lb}}{1}\right)\left(\frac{1 \text{ kg}}{2.2 \text{ lb}}\right)\left(\frac{2 \text{ mL}}{500 \text{ mg}}\right) = 5 \text{ mL}$$

29) Your 64 YO 152 lb, 5 ft 8 in female patient diagnosed with advanced bladder cancer has been prescribed ifosfamide 1500 mg/m²/day IV for 5 days. You calculate the BSA using the Mosteller method as being 1.82 m². Ifosfamide is available in 60 mL vials containing 3 g of drug. How many mL will you administer each day?

$$\frac{1500 \text{ mg}}{\text{m}^2 \text{ day}} \left(\frac{1.82 \text{ m}^2}{1}\right)\left(\frac{60 \text{ mL}}{3 \text{ g}}\right)\left(\frac{1 \text{ g}}{1000 \text{ mg}}\right) = \frac{54.6 \text{ mL}}{\text{day}}$$

30) A 16 YO is to receive cephalexin 250 mg PO q 6 h for 10 days. The drug is available in 250 mg capsules. How many capsules will the patient receive in the 10-day course of therapy?

$$10 \text{ days} \left(\frac{250 \text{ mg}}{\text{dose}}\right)\left(\frac{4 \text{ doses}}{\text{day}}\right)\left(\frac{1 \text{ cap}}{250 \text{ mg}}\right) = 40 \text{ caps}$$

Or just:

$$\frac{4 \text{ caps}}{\text{day}}\left(\frac{10 \text{ days}}{1}\right) = 40 \text{ caps}$$

Chapter 11
BSA Calculation Problems

Calculate the BSA in m² for the following individuals.

1) An adult female weighing 125 lb and 5 ft 7 in tall.

$$BSA = \sqrt{\frac{125 \times 67}{3131}} = 1.64 \text{ m}^2$$

2) A 6 YO boy weighing 21 kg and 116 cm tall.

$$BSA = \sqrt{\frac{21 \times 116}{3600}} = 0.82 \text{ m}^2$$

3) An adult male weighing 175 lb and 6 ft tall.

$$BSA = \sqrt{\frac{175 \times 72}{3131}} = 2.00 \text{ m}^2$$

4) A 13-month-old girl weighing 21 lb and 30 in tall.

$$BSA = \sqrt{\frac{21 \times 30}{3131}} = 0.45 \text{ m}^2$$

5) A 16 YO female weighing 53 kg and 161 cm tall.

$$BSA = \sqrt{\frac{53 \times 161}{3600}} = 1.54 \text{ m}^2$$

6) An adult female weighing 151 lb and 5 ft 1 in tall.

$$BSA = \sqrt{\frac{151 \times 61}{3131}} = 1.72 \text{ m}^2$$

7) An adult male weighing 242 lb and 6 ft 7 in tall.

$$BSA = \sqrt{\frac{242 \times 79}{3131}} = 2.47 \text{ m}^2$$

8) An adult male weighing 154 lb and 5 ft 10 in tall.

$$BSA = \sqrt{\frac{154 \times 70}{3131}} = 1.86 \text{ m}^2$$

9) An adult female weighing 50 kg and 4 ft 9 in tall.

4 ft 9 in = 57 in   57 in (2.54 cm/in) = 145 cm (Or you could convert the 50 kg to pounds and use the other formula.

$$BSA = \sqrt{\frac{50 \times 145}{3600}} = 1.42 \text{ m}^2$$

10) An adult male weighing 82 kg and 183 cm tall.

$$BSA = \sqrt{\frac{82 \times 183}{3600}} = 2.04 \text{ m}^2$$

Calculate the following:

11) A 49 YO male patient who weighs 170 lb and is 5 ft 11 in tall is being treated for refractory multiple myeloma and will be placed on a carfilzomib 20/27 mg/m² IV twice weekly regimen. Cycle 1 of the regimen will be 20 mg/m² infused over 10 minutes on days 1 and 2, followed by 27 mg/m² over 10 minutes on days 8, 9, 15, and 16 of a 28-day treatment cycle.

a) Calculate the patient's BSA.

$$BSA = \sqrt{\frac{170 \times 71}{3131}} = 1.96 \text{ m}^2$$

b) Calculate the dose in mg the patient will receive on days 1 and 2.

$$1.96 \text{ m}^2 \left(\frac{20 \text{ mg}}{\text{m}^2}\right) = 39.2 \text{ mg}$$

c) Calculate the dose the patient will receive on days 8, 9, 15, and 16.

$$1.96 \text{ m}^2 \left(\frac{27 \text{ mg}}{\text{m}^2}\right) = 52.9 \text{ mg}$$

12) A 68 YO male patient who weighs 155 lb and is 5 ft 9 in tall is being treated for acute myeloid leukemia with IV idarubicin 12 mg/m²/day for 3 days (in combination with cytarabine).

a) Calculate the patient's BSA.

$$BSA = \sqrt{\frac{155 \times 69}{3131}} = 1.85 \text{ m}^2$$

b) Calculate the daily dose in mg for this patient.

$$1.85 \text{ m}^2 \left(\frac{12 \text{ mg}}{\text{m}^2 \text{ day}}\right) = \frac{22.2 \text{ mg}}{\text{day}}$$

13) A 9 YO 64 lb boy who is 4 ft 5 in tall is to receive IV topotecan 2.4 mg/m² once daily for 7 days for treatment of acute lymphoblastic leukemia.

a) Calculate the patient's BSA.

$$BSA = \sqrt{\frac{64 \times 53}{3131}} = 1.04 \text{ m}^2$$

b) Calculate the daily dose in mg for this patient.

$$1.04 \text{ m}^2 \left(\frac{2.4 \text{ mg}}{\text{m}^2}\right) = 2.5 \text{ mg}$$

14) A 10 YO male child who weighs 32 kg and is 139 cm tall will start the BEACOPP regimen for treatment of Hodgkin lymphoma. Oral prednisone is part of the regimen dosed at 40 mg/m²/day in 2 divided doses on days 0 to 13.

a) Calculate the patient's BSA.

$$BSA = \sqrt{\frac{32 \times 139}{3600}} = 1.11 \text{ m}^2$$

b) How many milligrams of prednisone will the patient receive per dose?

$$1.11 \text{ m}^2 \left(\frac{40 \text{ mg}}{\text{m}^2 \text{ day}}\right)\left(\frac{1 \text{ day}}{2 \text{ doses}}\right) = \frac{22.2 \text{ mg}}{\text{dose}}$$

Chapter 12
Pediatric Dosing Problems

The recommended oral dosage of cephalexin to treat impetigo in infants, children and adolescents is 25 to 50 mg/kg/day divided every 6 to 8 hours (with a maximum dose of 250 mg/dose) for at least 7 days. A 15-month-old, 23 lb child has been prescribed 100 mg PO q 8 h for 7 days. The drug is available as 250 mg/5 mL.

1) What is the recommended range in mg/dose for this child when dosed q 8 h?

$$\frac{25 \text{ mg}}{\text{kg day}} \left(\frac{23 \text{ lb}}{1}\right)\left(\frac{1 \text{ kg}}{2.2 \text{ lb}}\right)\left(\frac{1 \text{ day}}{3 \text{ doses}}\right) = \frac{87 \text{ mg}}{\text{dose}}$$

$$\frac{50 \text{ mg}}{\text{kg day}} \left(\frac{23 \text{ lb}}{1}\right)\left(\frac{1 \text{ kg}}{2.2 \text{ lb}}\right)\left(\frac{1 \text{ day}}{3 \text{ doses}}\right) = \frac{174 \text{ mg}}{\text{dose}}$$

87 to 174 mg/dose

2) Is the prescribed dosage within the recommended range for impetigo?

Yes, 100 mg/dose is between 87 and 174 mg/dose.

3) What is the range in mL/dose for this child?

$$\frac{87 \text{ mg}}{\text{dose}}\left(\frac{5 \text{ mL}}{250 \text{ mg}}\right) = \frac{1.7 \text{ mL}}{\text{dose}}$$

$$\frac{174 \text{ mg}}{\text{dose}}\left(\frac{5 \text{ mL}}{250 \text{ mg}}\right) = \frac{3.5 \text{ mL}}{\text{dose}}$$

1.7 to 3.5 mL/dose

4) How many mL/dose would the child receive for the prescribed dosage?

$$\frac{100 \text{ mg}}{\text{dose}}\left(\frac{5 \text{ mL}}{250 \text{ mg}}\right) = \frac{2 \text{ mL}}{\text{dose}}$$

The recommended oral dosage of amoxicillin to treat acute otitis media (AOM) for infants (2 months and over) and children is 80 to 90 mg/kg/day in divided doses every 12 hours. The duration of therapy will vary with patient age and severity of symptoms. A 6-month-old infant weighing 18 lb has been prescribed 350 mg q 12 h. The drug is available as 250 mg/5 mL.

5) What is the recommended range in mg/dose for this child?

$$\frac{80 \text{ mg}}{\text{kg day}}\left(\frac{18 \text{ lb}}{1}\right)\left(\frac{1 \text{ kg}}{2.2 \text{ lb}}\right)\left(\frac{1 \text{ day}}{2 \text{ doses}}\right) = \frac{327 \text{ mg}}{\text{dose}}$$

$$\frac{90 \text{ mg}}{\text{kg day}}\left(\frac{18 \text{ lb}}{1}\right)\left(\frac{1 \text{ kg}}{2.2 \text{ lb}}\right)\left(\frac{1 \text{ day}}{2 \text{ doses}}\right) = \frac{368 \text{ mg}}{\text{dose}}$$

327 to 368 mg/dose

6) Is the prescribed dosage within the recommended range for AOM?

Yes, 350 mg/dose is between 327 and 368 mg/dose.

7) What is the recommended range in mL/dose for this child?

$$\frac{327 \text{ mg}}{\text{dose}} \left(\frac{5 \text{ mL}}{250 \text{ mg}}\right) = \frac{6.5 \text{ mL}}{\text{dose}}$$

$$\frac{368 \text{ mg}}{\text{dose}} \left(\frac{5 \text{ mL}}{250 \text{ mg}}\right) = \frac{7.4 \text{ mL}}{\text{dose}}$$

6.5 to 7.4 mL/dose

8) How many mL/dose would the child receive for the prescribed dosage?

$$\frac{350 \text{ mg}}{\text{dose}} \left(\frac{5 \text{ mL}}{250 \text{ mg}}\right) = \frac{7 \text{ mL}}{\text{dose}}$$

The recommended oral dosage for diphenhydramine is 5 mg/kg/day divided into 3-4 doses when treating allergies in infants, children and adolescents. A 6 YO 46 lb male child has been prescribed 25 mg PO q 6 h. Diphenhydramine is available as an oral solution containing 12.5 mg/5 mL.

9) Is this a reasonable dosage for this child?

$$\frac{5 \text{ mg}}{\text{kg day}} \left(\frac{46 \text{ lb}}{1}\right)\left(\frac{1 \text{ kg}}{2.2 \text{ lb}}\right)\left(\frac{1 \text{ day}}{4 \text{ doses}}\right) = \frac{26 \text{ mg}}{\text{dose}}$$

Yes. 25 mg/dose is just below the recommended dose of 26 mg/dose.

10) How many mL/dose will the child receive?

$$25 \text{ mg} \left(\frac{5 \text{ mL}}{12.5 \text{ mg}}\right) = 10 \text{ mL}$$

Azithromycin has several different oral regimens to treat OM in children six months and older. The 3-day regimen is 10 mg/kg once daily for 3 days (maximum: 500 mg/day). Azithromycin is available as 200 mg/5 mL.

11) How many mL would a 3 YO boy weighing 31 lb receive each day?

$$\frac{10 \text{ mg}}{\text{kg day}} \left(\frac{31 \text{ lb}}{1}\right)\left(\frac{1 \text{ kg}}{2.2 \text{ lb}}\right)\left(\frac{5 \text{ mL}}{200 \text{ mg}}\right) = \frac{3.5 \text{ mL}}{\text{day}}$$

The dosing guidelines for oral morphine sulfate solution for treating moderate to severe acute pain in infants >6 months, children and adolescents who are <50 kg is 0.2 to 0.5 mg/kg/dose every 3 to 4 hours as needed and for children and adolescents 50 kg and over it is 15 to 20 mg every 3 to 4 hours as needed. Morphine sulfate oral solution 2 mg/mL and 4 mg/mL is available.

12) Using the above information, what is the normal mg/dose range for a 7 YO 23 kg male child?

$$\frac{0.2 \text{ mg}}{\text{kg dose}} \left(\frac{23 \text{ kg}}{1}\right) = \frac{4.6 \text{ mg}}{\text{dose}}$$

$$\frac{0.5 \text{ mg}}{\text{kg dose}} \left(\frac{23 \text{ kg}}{1}\right) = \frac{11.5 \text{ mg}}{\text{dose}}$$

4.6 to 11.5 mg/dose

13) What is the normal mL/dose range using the 2 mg/mL solution for a 15-month-old 23 lb child?

$$\frac{0.2 \text{ mg}}{\text{kg dose}} \left(\frac{23 \text{ lb}}{1}\right)\left(\frac{1 \text{ kg}}{2.2 \text{ lb}}\right)\left(\frac{1 \text{ mL}}{2 \text{ mg}}\right) = \frac{1 \text{ mL}}{\text{dose}}$$

$$\frac{0.5 \text{ mg}}{\text{kg dose}} \left(\frac{23 \text{ lb}}{1}\right)\left(\frac{1 \text{ kg}}{2.2 \text{ lb}}\right)\left(\frac{1 \text{ mL}}{2 \text{ mg}}\right) = \frac{2.6 \text{ mL}}{\text{dose}}$$

1 mL to 2.6 mL/dose

14) The prescriber has ordered 2 mL/dose of the 4 mg/mL morphine sulfate solution for your 4 YO patient who weighs 17 kg. Is this dose within the dosing guidelines?

$$\frac{0.2 \text{ mg}}{\text{kg dose}} \left(\frac{17 \text{ kg}}{1}\right)\left(\frac{1 \text{ mL}}{4 \text{ mg}}\right) = \frac{0.85 \text{ mL}}{\text{dose}}$$

$$\frac{0.5 \text{ mg}}{\text{kg dose}} \left(\frac{17 \text{ kg}}{1}\right)\left(\frac{1 \text{ mL}}{4 \text{ mg}}\right) = \frac{2.1 \text{ mL}}{\text{dose}}$$

Yes, 2 mL/dose is between 0.85 and 2.1 mL/dose.

15) The prescriber, who wants to order the highest recommended dose of oral morphine sulfate solution for a 14 kg 3 YO child, has ordered 3.9 mL of the 4 mg/mL solution. Is this the correct dose? If not, what is a possible cause of the error?

$$\text{Maximum dose } \frac{0.5 \text{ mg}}{\text{kg dose}} \left(\frac{14 \text{ kg}}{1}\right)\left(\frac{1 \text{ mL}}{4 \text{ mg}}\right) = \frac{1.8 \text{ mL}}{\text{dose}}$$

No, 3.9 mL of the 4 mg/mL is above the maximum dose of 1.8 mL for this child. The prescriber may have used the child's weight in pounds rather than the weight in kg.

The general dosing guidelines for IV ampicillin in treating mild to moderate infections in infants, children and adolescents is 100 to 150 mg/kg/day divided every 6 hours with a maximum daily dose of 4000 mg. Using this information, answer the following questions.

16) What is the mg/dose range for a 9 YO 63 lb male child?

$$\frac{100 \text{ mg}}{\text{kg day}} \left(\frac{63 \text{ lb}}{1}\right)\left(\frac{1 \text{ kg}}{2.2 \text{ lb}}\right)\left(\frac{1 \text{ day}}{4 \text{ doses}}\right) = \frac{716 \text{ mg}}{\text{dose}}$$

$$\frac{150 \text{ mg}}{\text{kg day}} \left(\frac{63 \text{ lb}}{1}\right)\left(\frac{1 \text{ kg}}{2.2 \text{ lb}}\right)\left(\frac{1 \text{ day}}{4 \text{ doses}}\right) = \frac{1074 \text{ mg}}{\text{dose}}$$

1074 mg/dose exceeds the maximum of 1000 mg/dose. The range is 716 to 1000 mg/dose.

17) What is the mg/day range for a 6 YO 20 kg female child?

$$\frac{100 \text{ mg}}{\text{kg day}} \left(\frac{20 \text{ kg}}{1}\right) = \frac{2000 \text{ mg}}{\text{day}}$$

$$\frac{150 \text{ mg}}{\text{kg day}} \left(\frac{20 \text{ kg}}{1}\right) = \frac{3000 \text{ mg}}{\text{day}}$$

2000 to 3000 mg/day

18) The health care provider ordered 700 mg IV q 6 h for a 50 lb 7 YO female child.

a) Is this dosage within the general dosing guidelines?

$$\frac{100 \text{ mg}}{\text{kg day}} \left(\frac{50 \text{ lb}}{1}\right)\left(\frac{1 \text{ kg}}{2.2 \text{ lb}}\right)\left(\frac{1 \text{ day}}{4 \text{ doses}}\right) = \frac{568 \text{ mg}}{\text{dose}}$$

$$\frac{150 \text{ mg}}{\text{kg day}} \left(\frac{50 \text{ lb}}{1}\right)\left(\frac{1 \text{ kg}}{2.2 \text{ lb}}\right)\left(\frac{1 \text{ day}}{4 \text{ doses}}\right) = \frac{852 \text{ mg}}{\text{dose}}$$

Yes, 700 mg/dose is between 568 and 852 mg/dose.

b) How many mg/kg/day will this child be receiving?

$$\frac{700 \text{ mg}}{\text{dose}}\left(\frac{4 \text{ doses}}{\text{day}}\right)\left(\frac{1}{50 \text{ lb}}\right)\left(\frac{2.2 \text{ lb}}{\text{kg}}\right) = \frac{123 \text{ mg}}{\text{kg day}}$$

19) A 32 kg 10 YO female has been prescribed a dosage 140 mg/kg/day divided every 6 hours. Does this dosage fall within the general dosing guidelines?

Yes, 140 mg/kg/day is between 100 and 150 mg/kg/day.

Chapter 13
Pediatric Maintenance Fluid Replacement Calculations

Weight	24 Hour Fluid Requirement
Infants 3.5 to 10 kg	100 mL/kg
Children 11-20 kg	1000 mL + 50 mL/kg for every kg over 10
For children > 20 kg	1500 mL + 20 mL/kg for every kg over 20, up to a maximum of 2400 mL daily.

Use the above table in the following calculations. Round to the nearest mL and nearest mL/h.

1) Calculate the daily maintenance fluid requirement for an NPO child weighing 14 kg.

1000 mL + 4 kg (50 mL/kg) = 1000 mL + 200 mL = 1200 mL

2) Calculate the daily maintenance fluid requirement for an NPO child weighing 23 kg.

1500 mL + 3 kg (20 mL/kg) = 1500 mL + 60 mL = 1560 mL

3) Calculate the daily maintenance fluid requirement for an NPO child weighing 8.5 kg.

8.5 kg (100 mL/kg) = 850 mL

4) Calculate the daily maintenance fluid requirement for an NPO child weighing 41.5 kg.

1500 mL + 21.5 kg (20 mL/kg) = 1500 mL + 430 mL = 1930 mL

5) Calculate the infusion rate to the nearest mL/h to deliver daily maintenance fluids to an NPO child weighing 32 kg.

24 h fluid requirement = 1500 mL + 12 kg (20 mL/kg) = 1500 mL + 240 mL = 1740 mL

1740 mL/24 h = 73 mL/h

6) A 35 kg NPO child is on 70% fluid maintenance (70% of the calculated amount in the above table). At what rate will you set the infusion pump?

24 h fluid requirement = 1500 mL + 15 kg (20 mL/kg) = 1500 mL + 300 mL = 1800 mL

70% of 1800 mL = 1260 mL

1260 mL/24 h = 53 mL/h

7) What is the daily maintenance fluid requirement for an NPO child on 70% fluid maintenance who weighs 45 kg? At what rate will you set the infusion pump?

24 h fluid requirement = 1500 mL + 25 kg (20 mL/kg) = 1500 mL + 500 mL = 2000 mL

70% of 2000 mL = 1400 mL

1400 mL/24 h = 58 mL/h

8) What is the daily maintenance fluid requirement for an NPO child on 70% fluid maintenance who weighs 19.5 kg? At what rate will you set the infusion pump?

24 h fluid requirement = 1000 mL + 9.5 kg (50 mL/kg) = 1000 mL + 475 mL = 1475 mL

70% of 1475 mL = 1033 mL

1033 mL/24 h = 43 mL/h

9) At what rate will you set the infusion pump to deliver maintenance fluids to a 15 kg NPO child who is on 70% fluid maintenance?

24 h fluid requirement = 1000 mL + 5 kg (50 mL/kg) = 1000 mL + 250 mL = 1250 mL

70% of 1250 mL = 875 mL

875 mL/24 h = 36 mL/h

10) Calculate the daily maintenance fluid requirement for an NPO child weighing 28 kg.

1500 mL + 8 kg (20 mL/kg) = 1500 mL + 160 mL = 1660 mL

11) What is the daily maintenance fluid requirement for an NPO child on 70% fluid maintenance who weighs 36 kg?

24 h fluid requirement = 1500 mL + 16 kg (20 mL/kg) = 1500 mL + 320 mL = 1820 mL

70% of 1820 mL = 1274 mL

12) Calculate the daily maintenance fluid requirement for an NPO child weighing 31.5 kg.

1500 mL + 11.5 kg (20 mL/kg) = 1500 mL + 230 mL = 1730 mL

Chapter 14
IV Flow Rate Calculations Level I

Round all drops/min calculations to the nearest drop and all mL/h calculations to the nearest tenth mL/h.

Calculate the flow rate in mL/h.

1) 1000 mL infused over 4 hours.

$$\frac{1000 \text{ mL}}{4 \text{ h}} = \frac{250 \text{ mL}}{\text{h}}$$

2) 500 mL infused over 6 hours.

$$\frac{500 \text{ mL}}{6 \text{ h}} = \frac{83.3 \text{ mL}}{\text{h}}$$

3) 1000 mL infused over 8 hours.

$$\frac{1000 \text{ mL}}{8 \text{ h}} = \frac{125 \text{ mL}}{\text{h}}$$

4) 500 mL infused over 3 hours.

$$\frac{500 \text{ mL}}{3 \text{ h}} = \frac{166.7 \text{ mL}}{\text{h}}$$

5) 1000 mL infused over 5 hours.

$$\frac{1000 \text{ mL}}{5 \text{ h}} = \frac{200 \text{ mL}}{\text{h}}$$

6) 250 mL infused over 90 minutes.

$$\frac{250 \text{ mL}}{90 \text{ min}} \left(\frac{60 \text{ min}}{\text{h}}\right) = \frac{166.7 \text{ mL}}{\text{h}}$$

Or

$$\frac{250 \text{ mL}}{1.5 \text{ h}} = \frac{166.7 \text{ mL}}{\text{h}}$$

7) 500 mL infused over 4 hours 15 minutes.

$$\frac{500 \text{ mL}}{4.25 \text{ h}} = \frac{117.6 \text{ mL}}{\text{h}}$$

8) 1000 mL infused over 6 hours 30 minutes.

$$\frac{1000 \text{ mL}}{6.5 \text{ h}} = \frac{153.8 \text{ mL}}{\text{h}}$$

9) 250 mL infused over 45 minutes.

$$\frac{250 \text{ mL}}{45 \text{ min}} \left(\frac{60 \text{ min}}{\text{h}}\right) = \frac{333.3 \text{ mL}}{\text{h}}$$

Or

$$\frac{250 \text{ mL}}{0.75 \text{ h}} = \frac{333.3 \text{ mL}}{\text{h}}$$

10) 500 mL infused over 3 hours 15 minutes.

$$\frac{500 \text{ mL}}{3.25 \text{ h}} = \frac{153.8 \text{ mL}}{\text{h}}$$

Calculate the flow rate in drops/min.

11) 1000 mL infused over 5 hours with a drop factor of 20 (20 gtts/mL).

$$\frac{1000 \text{ mL}}{5 \text{ h}} \left(\frac{1 \text{ h}}{60 \text{ min}}\right)\left(\frac{20 \text{ gtts}}{\text{mL}}\right) = \frac{67 \text{ gtts}}{\text{min}}$$

12) 1000 mL infused over 6 hours with a drop factor of 15 (15 gtts/mL).

$$\frac{1000 \text{ mL}}{6 \text{ h}} \left(\frac{1 \text{ h}}{60 \text{ min}}\right)\left(\frac{15 \text{ gtts}}{\text{mL}}\right) = \frac{42 \text{ gtts}}{\text{min}}$$

13) 250 mL infused over 2 hours with a microdrip set (60 gtts/mL).

$$\frac{250 \text{ mL}}{2 \text{ h}} \left(\frac{1 \text{ h}}{60 \text{ min}}\right)\left(\frac{60 \text{ gtts}}{\text{mL}}\right) = \frac{125 \text{ gtts}}{\text{min}}$$

14) 500 mL infused over 7 hours with a drop factor of 10.

$$\frac{500 \text{ mL}}{7 \text{ h}} \left(\frac{1 \text{ h}}{60 \text{ min}}\right)\left(\frac{10 \text{ gtts}}{\text{mL}}\right) = \frac{12 \text{ gtts}}{\text{min}}$$

15) 100 mL infused over 1 h with a drop factor of 15.

$$\frac{100 \text{ mL}}{\text{h}} \left(\frac{1 \text{ h}}{60 \text{ min}}\right)\left(\frac{15 \text{ gtts}}{\text{mL}}\right) = \frac{25 \text{ gtts}}{\text{min}}$$

16) 500 mL infused over 4 hours with a drop factor of 20.

$$\frac{500 \text{ mL}}{4 \text{ h}} \left(\frac{1 \text{ h}}{60 \text{ min}}\right)\left(\frac{20 \text{ gtts}}{\text{mL}}\right) = \frac{42 \text{ gtts}}{\text{min}}$$

17) 500 mL infused over 90 minutes with a drop factor of 10.

$$\frac{500 \text{ mL}}{90 \text{ min}} \left(\frac{10 \text{ gtts}}{\text{mL}}\right) = \frac{56 \text{ gtts}}{\text{min}}$$

18) 1000 mL infused over 3 hours 30 minutes with a drop factor of 15.

$$\frac{1000 \text{ mL}}{3.5 \text{ h}} \left(\frac{1 \text{ h}}{60 \text{ min}}\right)\left(\frac{15 \text{ gtts}}{\text{mL}}\right) = \frac{71 \text{ gtts}}{\text{min}}$$

19) 1000 mL infused over 10 hours 15 minutes with a drop factor of 60.

$$\frac{1000 \text{ mL}}{10.25 \text{ h}} \left(\frac{1 \text{ h}}{60 \text{ min}}\right)\left(\frac{60 \text{ gtts}}{\text{mL}}\right) = \frac{98 \text{ gtts}}{\text{min}}$$

20) 750 mL infused over 4 hours 20 minutes with a drop factor of 15.

$$\frac{750 \text{ mL}}{4.33 \text{ h}} \left(\frac{1 \text{ h}}{60 \text{ min}}\right)\left(\frac{15 \text{ gtts}}{\text{mL}}\right) = \frac{43 \text{ gtts}}{\text{min}}$$

Calculate the length of time in hours and minutes, rounded to the nearest minute, required to infuse the following:

21) 1000 mL at 90 mL/h.

$$1000 \text{ mL} \left(\frac{1 \text{ h}}{90 \text{ mL}}\right) = 11.11 \text{ h} = 11 \text{ h } 7 \text{ min}$$

Note: 0.11 h (60 min/h) = 6.6 min rounded to 7 min.

22) 500 mL at 125 mL/h.

$$500 \text{ mL} \left(\frac{1 \text{ h}}{125 \text{ mL}}\right) = 4 \text{ h}$$

23) 100 mL at 64 mL/h.

$$100 \text{ mL} \left(\frac{1 \text{ h}}{64 \text{ mL}}\right) = 1.56 \text{ h} = 1 \text{ h } 34 \text{ min}$$

24) 250 mL at 31 gtts/min with a drop factor of 20.

$$250 \text{ mL} \left(\frac{1 \text{ min}}{31 \text{ gtts}}\right)\left(\frac{20 \text{ gtts}}{\text{mL}}\right) = 161 \text{ min} = 2 \text{ h } 41 \text{ min}$$

Note: 2 h = 120 min. 161 min - 120 min = 41 min

25) 500 mL at 43 gtts/min with a drop factor of 10.

$$500 \text{ mL} \left(\frac{1 \text{ min}}{43 \text{ gtts}}\right)\left(\frac{10 \text{ gtts}}{\text{mL}}\right) = 116 \text{ min} = 1 \text{ h } 56 \text{ min}$$

26) 1000 mL at 50 gtts/min with a drop factor of 15.

$$1000 \text{ mL} \left(\frac{1 \text{ min}}{50 \text{ gtts}}\right)\left(\frac{15 \text{ gtts}}{\text{mL}}\right) = 300 \text{ min} = 5 \text{ h}$$

27) 500 mL at 24 gtts/min with a drop factor of 20.

$$500 \text{ mL} \left(\frac{1 \text{ min}}{24 \text{ gtts}}\right)\left(\frac{20 \text{ gtts}}{\text{mL}}\right) = 417 \text{ min} = 6 \text{ h } 57 \text{ min}$$

28) 1000 mL at 60 gtts/min with a drop factor of 10.

$$1000 \text{ mL} \left(\frac{1 \text{ min}}{60 \text{ gtts}}\right)\left(\frac{10 \text{ gtts}}{\text{mL}}\right) = 167 \text{ min} = 2 \text{ h } 47 \text{ min}$$

29) 500 mL at 25 mL/h.

$$500 \text{ mL} \left(\frac{1 \text{ h}}{25 \text{ mL}}\right) = 20 \text{ h}$$

30) 1000 mL at 60 mL/h.

$$1000 \text{ mL} \left(\frac{1 \text{ h}}{60 \text{ mL}}\right) = 16.67 \text{ h} = 16 \text{ h } 40 \text{ min}$$

Calculate the volume infused in the following scenarios. Round to the nearest mL.

31) Infusion rate of 40 mL/h for 3 hours 15 min.

$$3.25 \text{ h} \left(\frac{40 \text{ mL}}{\text{h}}\right) = 130 \text{ mL}$$

32) Infusion rate of 65 mL/h for 2 hours 30 min.

$$2.5\,h\left(\frac{65\,mL}{h}\right) = 163\,mL$$

33) Infusion rate of 24 gtts/min, drop factor 20, for 4 hours 20 min.

$$4.33\,h\left(\frac{24\,gtts}{min}\right)\left(\frac{60\,min}{h}\right)\left(\frac{1\,mL}{20\,gtts}\right) = 312\,mL$$

34) Infusion rate of 72 gtts/min, drop factor 15, for 6 hours 15 min.

$$6.25\,h\left(\frac{72\,gtts}{min}\right)\left(\frac{60\,min}{h}\right)\left(\frac{1\,mL}{15\,gtts}\right) = 1800\,mL$$

35) Infusion rate of 32 mL/h for 3 h 10 minutes.

$$3.17\,h\left(\frac{32\,mL}{h}\right) = 101\,mL$$

36) Infusion rate of 45 gtts/min, drop factor 20, for 6 hours 15 min.

$$6.25\,h\left(\frac{45\,gtts}{min}\right)\left(\frac{60\,min}{h}\right)\left(\frac{1\,mL}{20\,gtts}\right) = 844\,mL$$

37) Infusion rate of 30 mL per hour for 4 hours 30 min.

$$4.5\,h\left(\frac{30\,mL}{h}\right) = 135\,mL$$

38) Infusion rate of 62 mL per hour for 1 hour 15 min.

$$1.25\,h\left(\frac{62\,mL}{h}\right) = 78\,mL$$

39) Infusion rate of 34 mL/h for 90 min.

$$1.5\,h\left(\frac{34\,mL}{h}\right) = 51\,mL$$

40) Infusion rate of 45 gtts/min, drop factor 20, for 6 hours 20 min.

$$6.33\,h\left(\frac{45\,gtts}{min}\right)\left(\frac{60\,min}{h}\right)\left(\frac{1\,mL}{20\,gtts}\right) = 855\,mL$$

Chapter 15
IV Flow Rate Calculations Level 2

Round all drops/min to the nearest drop. Round all mL/hour rates for the infusion pump to the nearest tenth mL/hour.

1) A healthcare provider has ordered dobutamine 10 mcg/kg/min IV for your 68 YO patient who weighs 172 lb. The dobutamine is available as 1000 mg/250 mL. At what rate will you set the IV infusion pump?

$$\frac{10 \text{ mcg}}{\text{kg min}} \left(\frac{172 \text{ lb}}{1}\right) \left(\frac{1 \text{ kg}}{2.2 \text{ lb}}\right) \left(\frac{250 \text{ mL}}{1000 \text{ mg}}\right) \left(\frac{1 \text{ mg}}{1000 \text{ mcg}}\right) \left(\frac{60 \text{ min}}{\text{h}}\right) = \frac{11.7 \text{ mL}}{\text{h}}$$

2) Mrs. Robinson, who has been diagnosed with acute decompensated heart failure, has an order for nitroglycerin 10 mcg/min IV. Mrs. Robinson weighs 142 lb. The NTG is available as 100 mg/250 mL. At what rate will you set the IV infusion pump?

$$\frac{10 \text{ mcg}}{\text{min}} \left(\frac{250 \text{ mL}}{100 \text{ mg}}\right) \left(\frac{1 \text{ mg}}{1000 \text{ mcg}}\right) \left(\frac{60 \text{ min}}{\text{h}}\right) = \frac{1.5 \text{ mL}}{\text{h}}$$

3) A 170 lb patient has an order for dopamine 15 mcg/kg/min to treat heart failure. The courteous pharmacy staff sends a 250 mL bag labeled dopamine 3200 mcg/mL. At what rate will you set the IV infusion pump?

$$\frac{15 \text{ mcg}}{\text{kg min}} \left(\frac{170 \text{ lb}}{1}\right) \left(\frac{1 \text{ kg}}{2.2 \text{ lb}}\right) \left(\frac{1 \text{ mL}}{3200 \text{ mcg}}\right) \left(\frac{60 \text{ min}}{\text{h}}\right) = \frac{21.7 \text{ mL}}{\text{h}}$$

4) Your 81 kg patient has an order for dobutamine 15 mcg/kg/min IV to start at 0900. The dobutamine is available as 500 mg in 250 mL D5W. At what rate will you set the IV infusion pump?

$$\frac{15 \text{ mcg}}{\text{kg min}} \left(\frac{81 \text{ kg}}{1}\right) \left(\frac{250 \text{ mL}}{500 \text{ mg}}\right) \left(\frac{1 \text{ mg}}{1000 \text{ mcg}}\right) \left(\frac{60 \text{ min}}{\text{h}}\right) = \frac{36.5 \text{ mL}}{\text{h}}$$

5) Your 67 YO 74 kg patient has an order for a lidocaine infusion at the rate of 20 mcg/kg/min. You have a 250 mL bag labeled "Lidocaine HCl and 5% Dextrose Injection USP". Lidocaine 2 g (8 mg/mL) is printed in big red letters in the middle of the label. What rate will you set the IV infusion pump?

$$\frac{20 \text{ mcg}}{\text{kg min}} \left(\frac{74 \text{ kg}}{1}\right) \left(\frac{1 \text{ mL}}{1000 \text{ mg}}\right) \left(\frac{1 \text{ mg}}{8 \text{ mg}}\right) \left(\frac{1 \text{ mg}}{1000 \text{ mcg}}\right) \left(\frac{60 \text{ min}}{\text{h}}\right) = \frac{11.1 \text{ mL}}{\text{h}}$$

6) Your 71 kg patient is receiving a dopamine infusion at the rate of 14 mL/h. The dopamine is mixed as 200 mg of dopamine in 250 mL of D5W. The infusion has been running for 1 hour 45 minutes. How many mcg/kg/min is the patient receiving?

$$\frac{14 \text{ mL}}{\text{h}} \left(\frac{200 \text{ mg}}{250 \text{ mL}}\right) \left(\frac{1 \text{ h}}{60 \text{ min}}\right) \left(\frac{1}{71 \text{ kg}}\right) \left(\frac{1000 \text{ mcg}}{\text{mg}}\right) = \frac{2.6 \text{ mcg}}{\text{kg min}}$$

7) A 38 YO female weighing 125 lb who is being treated for a bite wound infection has an order for ciprofloxacin 400 mg IV every 12 hours to be infused by slow IV infusion over 60 minutes. Ciprofloxacin is available in 200 mL bags containing 400 mg. You are using an IV administration set with a drop factor of 20. How many drops/min will you administer?

$$\frac{400 \text{ mg}}{60 \text{ min}} \left(\frac{200 \text{ mL}}{400 \text{ mg}}\right) \left(\frac{20 \text{ gtts}}{\text{mL}}\right) = \frac{67 \text{ gtts}}{\text{min}}$$

8) Your 140 lb, 5 ft 4 in female patient has an order for dobutamine 5 mcg/kg/min IV to start at 1400. The dobutamine is available as 1000 mcg/mL. At what rate will you set the IV infusion pump?

$$\frac{5 \text{ mcg}}{\text{kg min}} \left(\frac{140 \text{ lb}}{1}\right) \left(\frac{1 \text{ kg}}{2.2 \text{ lb}}\right) \left(\frac{1 \text{ mL}}{1000 \text{ mcg}}\right) \left(\frac{60 \text{ min}}{\text{h}}\right) = \frac{19.1 \text{ mL}}{\text{h}}$$

9) Your 180 lb patient in vasodilatory shock has been ordered vasopressin 0.03 units/min IV. The vasopressin is available as 20 units/100 mL. At what rate will you set the IV infusion pump?

$$\frac{0.03 \text{ units}}{\text{min}} \left(\frac{100 \text{ mL}}{20 \text{ units}}\right) \left(\frac{60 \text{ min}}{h}\right) = \frac{9 \text{ mL}}{h}$$

10) A physician has ordered dobutamine 4 mcg/kg/min IV for your 57 YO patient who weighs 75 kg. The dobutamine is available as 1000 mg in 250 mL D5W. At what rate will you set the IV infusion pump?

$$\frac{4 \text{ mcg}}{\text{kg min}} \left(\frac{75 \text{ kg}}{1}\right) \left(\frac{250 \text{ mL}}{1000 \text{ mg}}\right) \left(\frac{1 \text{ mg}}{1000 \text{ mcg}}\right) \left(\frac{60 \text{ min}}{h}\right) = \frac{4.5 \text{ mL}}{h}$$

11) A 52 YO female who weighs 76 kg is to receive vancomycin 2 g in 400 mL D5W at a rate of 10 mg/min. At what rate will you set the IV infusion pump?

$$\frac{10 \text{ mg}}{\text{min}} \left(\frac{400 \text{ mL}}{2 \text{ g}}\right) \left(\frac{1 \text{ g}}{1000 \text{ mg}}\right) \left(\frac{60 \text{ min}}{h}\right) = \frac{120 \text{ mL}}{h}$$

12) A 57 YO male weighing 165 lb, who has been diagnosed with meningitis, has an order for gentamicin 5 mg/kg/day in 3 divided doses. Each dose is to be administered over 120 minutes. The drug is available in 100 mL bags containing 125 mg. At what rate will you set the IV infusion pump?

$$\frac{5 \text{ mg}}{\text{kg day}} \left(\frac{165 \text{ lb}}{1}\right) \left(\frac{1 \text{ kg}}{2.2 \text{ lb}}\right) \left(\frac{1 \text{ day}}{3 \text{ doses}}\right) \left(\frac{1 \text{ dose}}{120 \text{ min}}\right) \left(\frac{100 \text{ mL}}{125 \text{ mg}}\right) \left(\frac{60 \text{ min}}{h}\right) = \frac{50 \text{ mL}}{h}$$

(You might want to break this on up into smaller pieces.)

13) Mr. Dombroski, who has been diagnosed with acute decompensated heart failure, has an order for nitroglycerin 15 mcg/min IV. Mr. Dombroski weighs 195 lb and is 6 ft 1 in tall. The NTG is available as 100 mg/250 mL. At what rate will you set the IV infusion pump?

$$\frac{15 \text{ mcg}}{\text{min}} \left(\frac{250 \text{ mL}}{100 \text{ mg}}\right) \left(\frac{1 \text{ mg}}{1000 \text{ mcg}}\right) \left(\frac{60 \text{ min}}{h}\right) = \frac{2.3 \text{ mL}}{h}$$

14) Your 55 kg patient is experiencing angina and has an order for nitroglycerin 5 mcg/min IV. The NTG is available as 100 mg/250 mL. At what rate will you set the IV infusion pump?

$$\frac{5 \text{ mcg}}{\text{min}} \left(\frac{250 \text{ mL}}{100 \text{ mg}}\right) \left(\frac{1 \text{ mg}}{1000 \text{ mcg}}\right) \left(\frac{60 \text{ min}}{h}\right) = \frac{0.8 \text{ mL}}{h}$$

15) You are starting your 174 lb patient on a lidocaine infusion at the rate of 20 mcg/kg/min. You have a 500 mL bag labeled "Lidocaine HCl and 5% Dextrose Injection USP". Lidocaine 2 g (4 mg/mL) is printed in big red letters in the middle of the label. What rate will you set the IV infusion pump?

$$\frac{20 \text{ mcg}}{\text{kg min}} \left(\frac{174 \text{ lb}}{1}\right) \left(\frac{1 \text{ kg}}{2.2 \text{ lb}}\right) \left(\frac{1 \text{ mL}}{4 \text{ mg}}\right) \left(\frac{1 \text{ mg}}{1000 \text{ mcg}}\right) \left(\frac{60 \text{ min}}{h}\right) = \frac{23.7 \text{ mL}}{h}$$

16) A 21 lb, 10-month-old infant, in shock has an order for norepinephrine 0.1 mcg/kg/min IV. The norepinephrine is available in a concentration of 8 mcg/mL. At what rate will you set the IV infusion pump?

$$\frac{0.1 \text{ mcg}}{\text{kg min}} \left(\frac{21 \text{ lb}}{1}\right) \left(\frac{1 \text{ kg}}{2.2 \text{ lb}}\right) \left(\frac{1 \text{ mL}}{8 \text{ mcg}}\right) \left(\frac{60 \text{ min}}{h}\right) = \frac{7.2 \text{ mL}}{h}$$

17) Your 55 YO female patient, who has been diagnosed with septic shock, weighs 155 lb. She has an order for norepinephrine 0.1 mcg/kg/min IV. The pharmacy delivers a bag containing 4 mg norepinephrine in 250 mL D5NS. At what rate will you set the IV infusion pump?

$$\frac{0.1 \text{ mcg}}{\text{kg min}} \left(\frac{155 \text{ lb}}{1}\right) \left(\frac{1 \text{ kg}}{2.2 \text{ lb}}\right) \left(\frac{250 \text{ mL}}{4 \text{ mg}}\right) \left(\frac{1 \text{ mg}}{1000 \text{ mcg}}\right) \left(\frac{60 \text{ min}}{h}\right) = \frac{26.4 \text{ mL}}{h}$$

18) A 55 YO male weighing 60 kg is to receive tobramycin 2 mg/kg/dose IV every 8 hours for a severe infection. Each dose will be administered over 40 minutes.

a) How many mg will the patient receive each dose?

$$\frac{2 \text{ mg}}{\text{kg dose}} \left(\frac{60 \text{ kg}}{1}\right) = \frac{120 \text{ mg}}{\text{dose}}$$

b) The pharmacy sends over the appropriate dose of tobramycin in a 100 mL bag of NS. At what rate will you set the IV infusion pump?

$$\frac{100 \text{ mL}}{40 \text{ min}} \left(\frac{60 \text{ min}}{\text{h}}\right) = \frac{150 \text{ mL}}{\text{h}}$$

19) Your 130 lb female patient has an order for dobutamine 5 mcg/kg/min IV to start at 1200. The dobutamine is available as 1000 mcg/mL. At what rate will you set the IV infusion pump?

$$\frac{5 \text{ mcg}}{\text{kg min}} \left(\frac{130 \text{ lb}}{1}\right) \left(\frac{1 \text{ kg}}{2.2 \text{ lb}}\right) \left(\frac{1 \text{ mL}}{1000 \text{ mcg}}\right) \left(\frac{60 \text{ min}}{\text{h}}\right) = \frac{17.7 \text{ mL}}{\text{h}}$$

20) A patient who weighs 175 lb is suffering from acute hypertension and has an order to start an infusion of nitroprusside 0.4 mcg/kg/min. The pharmacy delivers a 1000 mL bag containing 50 mg nitroprusside in D5W. At what rate will you set the IV infusion pump?

$$\frac{0.4 \text{ mcg}}{\text{kg min}} \left(\frac{175 \text{ lb}}{1}\right) \left(\frac{1 \text{ kg}}{2.2 \text{ lb}}\right) \left(\frac{1000 \text{ mL}}{50 \text{ mg}}\right) \left(\frac{1 \text{ mg}}{1000 \text{ mcg}}\right) \left(\frac{60 \text{ min}}{\text{h}}\right) = \frac{38.2 \text{ mL}}{\text{h}}$$

21) A 190 lb patient is receiving a 4 mg/mL lidocaine infusion at the rate of 24 mL/h. How many mcg/kg/min is the patient receiving?

$$\frac{24 \text{ mL}}{\text{h}} \left(\frac{4 \text{ mg}}{\text{mL}}\right) \left(\frac{1 \text{ h}}{60 \text{ min}}\right) \left(\frac{1}{190 \text{ lb}}\right) \left(\frac{2.2 \text{ lb}}{\text{kg}}\right) \left(\frac{1000 \text{ mcg}}{\text{mg}}\right) = \frac{18.5 \text{ mcg}}{\text{kg min}}$$

22) Your 95 kg patient is receiving a dopamine infusion at the rate of 15 mL/h. The dopamine is mixed as 200 mg of dopamine in 250 mL of D5W. The infusion has been running for 1 hour 25 minutes. How many mcg/kg/min is the patient receiving?

$$\frac{15 \text{ mL}}{\text{h}} \left(\frac{200 \text{ mg}}{250 \text{ mL}}\right) \left(\frac{1 \text{ h}}{60 \text{ min}}\right) \left(\frac{1}{95 \text{ kg}}\right) \left(\frac{1000 \text{ mcg}}{\text{mg}}\right) = \frac{2.1 \text{ mcg}}{\text{kg min}}$$

23) Your 60 kg patient has an order for dobutamine 10 mcg/kg/min IV to start at 1100. The dobutamine is available as 500 mg in 250 mL D5W. At what rate will you set the IV infusion pump?

$$\frac{10 \text{ mcg}}{\text{kg min}} \left(\frac{60 \text{ kg}}{1}\right) \left(\frac{250 \text{ mL}}{500 \text{ mg}}\right) \left(\frac{1 \text{ mg}}{1000 \text{ mcg}}\right) \left(\frac{60 \text{ min}}{\text{h}}\right) = \frac{18 \text{ mL}}{\text{h}}$$

24) Your 160 lb patient in vasodilatory shock has had his vasopressin titrated up to 0.035 units/min IV. The vasopressin is available as 20 units/100 mL. What rate will you set the IV infusion pump?

$$\frac{0.035 \text{ units}}{\text{min}} \left(\frac{100 \text{ mL}}{20 \text{ units}}\right) \left(\frac{60 \text{ min}}{\text{h}}\right) = \frac{10.5 \text{ mL}}{\text{h}}$$

25) Your 65 kg patient in septic shock has been ordered norepinephrine 1.5 mcg/kg/min IV. The norepinephrine is available as 4 mg in 250 mL D5W. What rate will you set the IV infusion pump?

$$\frac{1.5 \text{ mcg}}{\text{kg min}} \left(\frac{65 \text{ kg}}{1}\right) \left(\frac{250 \text{ mL}}{4 \text{ mg}}\right) \left(\frac{1 \text{ mg}}{1000 \text{ mcg}}\right) \left(\frac{60 \text{ min}}{\text{h}}\right) = \frac{365.6 \text{ mL}}{\text{h}}$$

26) A 77 kg patient is receiving a 4 mg/mL lidocaine infusion at the rate of 18 mL/h. How many mcg/kg/min is the patient receiving?

$$\frac{18 \text{ mL}}{\text{h}} \left(\frac{4 \text{ mg}}{\text{mL}}\right)\left(\frac{1 \text{ h}}{60 \text{ min}}\right)\left(\frac{1}{77 \text{ kg}}\right)\left(\frac{1000 \text{ mcg}}{\text{mg}}\right) = \frac{15.6 \text{ mcg}}{\text{kg min}}$$

27) A 9 kg, 8-month-old infant, in shock has an order for norepinephrine 0.05 mcg/kg/min IV. The norepinephrine is available in a concentration of 8 mcg/mL. At what rate will you set the IV infusion pump?

$$\frac{0.05 \text{ mcg}}{\text{kg min}}\left(\frac{9 \text{ kg}}{1}\right)\left(\frac{1 \text{ mL}}{8 \text{ mcg}}\right)\left(\frac{60 \text{ min}}{\text{h}}\right) = \frac{3.4 \text{ mL}}{\text{h}}$$

28) A 49 YO male who weighs 45 kg is to receive IV vancomycin 1 g in 200 mL D5W at a rate of 10 mg/min. At what rate will you set the IV infusion pump?

$$\frac{10 \text{ mg}}{\text{min}}\left(\frac{200 \text{ mL}}{1 \text{ g}}\right)\left(\frac{1 \text{ g}}{1000 \text{ mg}}\right)\left(\frac{60 \text{ min}}{\text{h}}\right) = \frac{120 \text{ mL}}{\text{h}}$$

29) A 67 YO male weighing 80 kg, who has been diagnosed with endocarditis, has an order for gentamicin 3 mg/kg/day IV in 2 divided doses. Each dose is to be administered over 120 minutes. The drug is available in 100 mL bags containing 120 mg. At what rate will you set the IV infusion pump?

$$\frac{3 \text{ mg}}{\text{kg day}}\left(\frac{80 \text{ kg}}{1}\right)\left(\frac{1 \text{ day}}{2 \text{ doses}}\right)\left(\frac{1 \text{ dose}}{120 \text{ min}}\right)\left(\frac{100 \text{ mL}}{120 \text{ mg}}\right)\left(\frac{60 \text{ min}}{\text{h}}\right) = \frac{50 \text{ mL}}{\text{h}}$$

30) Your 142 lb patient is experiencing angina and has had his IV nitroglycerin titrated up to 15 mcg/min. The NTG is available as 100 mg/250 mL. At what rate will you set the IV infusion pump?

$$\frac{15 \text{ mcg}}{\text{min}}\left(\frac{250 \text{ mL}}{100 \text{ mg}}\right)\left(\frac{1 \text{ mg}}{1000 \text{ mcg}}\right)\left(\frac{60 \text{ min}}{\text{h}}\right) = \frac{2.3 \text{ mL}}{\text{h}}$$

31) A 38 YO female weighing 125 lb, who is being treated for a bite wound infection, has an order for ciprofloxacin 400 mg IV every 12 hours to be infused by slow IV infusion over 60 minutes. Ciprofloxacin is available in 200 mL bags containing 400 mg. You are using an IV administration set with a drop factor of 10. How many drops/min will you administer?

$$\frac{400 \text{ mg}}{60 \text{ min}}\left(\frac{200 \text{ mL}}{400 \text{ mg}}\right)\left(\frac{10 \text{ gtts}}{\text{mL}}\right) = \frac{33 \text{ gtts}}{\text{min}}$$

32) An 84 kg patient has an order for dopamine 10 mcg/kg/min IV to treat cardiogenic shock. The pharmacy sends a 500 mL bag labeled dopamine 1600 mcg/mL. At what rate will you set the IV infusion pump?

$$\frac{10 \text{ mcg}}{\text{kg min}}\left(\frac{84 \text{ kg}}{1}\right)\left(\frac{1 \text{ mL}}{1600 \text{ mcg}}\right)\left(\frac{60 \text{ min}}{\text{h}}\right) = \frac{31.5 \text{ mL}}{\text{h}}$$

33) Your 45 YO female patient, who has been diagnosed with septic shock, weighs 67 kg. She has an order for norepinephrine 0.1 mcg/kg/min IV. The pharmacy delivers a bag containing 4 mg norepinephrine in 250 mL D5NS. At what rate will you set the IV infusion pump?

$$\frac{0.1 \text{ mcg}}{\text{kg min}}\left(\frac{67 \text{ kg}}{1}\right)\left(\frac{250 \text{ mL}}{4 \text{ mg}}\right)\left(\frac{1 \text{ mg}}{1000 \text{ mcg}}\right)\left(\frac{60 \text{ min}}{\text{h}}\right) = \frac{25.1 \text{ mL}}{\text{h}}$$

34) H.M., a 70 YO female weighing 68 kg with heart failure has an order for a continuous IV infusion of milrinone 0.5 mcg/kg/min. Milrinone is available in 100 mL bags containing 20 mg. At what rate will you set the IV infusion pump?

$$\frac{0.5 \text{ mcg}}{\text{kg min}}\left(\frac{68 \text{ kg}}{1}\right)\left(\frac{100 \text{ mL}}{20 \text{ mg}}\right)\left(\frac{1 \text{ mg}}{1000 \text{ mcg}}\right)\left(\frac{60 \text{ min}}{\text{h}}\right) = \frac{10.2 \text{ mL}}{\text{h}}$$

35) Your 65 kg 68 YO patient diagnosed with bradycardia has an order for epinephrine 0.4 mcg/kg/min IV. The pharmacy sends over a bag containing 1 mg epinephrine in 250 mL NS. At what rate will you set the IV infusion pump?

$$\frac{0.4 \text{ mcg}}{\text{kg min}} \left(\frac{65 \text{ kg}}{1}\right) \left(\frac{250 \text{ mL}}{1 \text{ mg}}\right) \left(\frac{1 \text{ mg}}{1000 \text{ mcg}}\right) \left(\frac{60 \text{ min}}{\text{h}}\right) = \frac{390 \text{ mL}}{\text{h}}$$

36) A patient who weighs 74 kg is suffering from acute hypertension and has an order to start an infusion of nitroprusside 0.5 mcg/kg/min. The pharmacy delivers a 1000 mL bag containing 50 mg nitroprusside in D5W. At what rate will you set the IV infusion pump?

$$\frac{0.5 \text{ mcg}}{\text{kg min}} \left(\frac{74 \text{ kg}}{1}\right) \left(\frac{1000 \text{ mL}}{50 \text{ mg}}\right) \left(\frac{1 \text{ mg}}{1000 \text{ mcg}}\right) \left(\frac{60 \text{ min}}{\text{h}}\right) = \frac{44.4 \text{ mL}}{\text{h}}$$

37) A 45 YO male weighing 65 kg is to receive tobramycin 2.5 mg/kg/dose IV every 12 hours for a severe infection. Each dose will be administered over 60 minutes.

a) How many mg will the patient receive each dose?

$$\frac{2.5 \text{ mg}}{\text{kg dose}} \left(\frac{65 \text{ kg}}{1}\right) = \frac{162.5 \text{ mg}}{\text{dose}}$$

b) The pharmacy sends over the appropriate dose of tobramycin in a 100 mL bag of NS. At what rate will you set the IV infusion pump?

$$\frac{100 \text{ mL}}{60 \text{ min}} \left(\frac{60 \text{ min}}{\text{h}}\right) = \frac{100 \text{ mL}}{\text{h}}$$

38) Your 64 kg patient in septic shock has been ordered norepinephrine 2 mcg/kg/min IV. The norepinephrine is available as 4 mg in 250 mL D5W. What rate will you set the IV infusion pump?

$$\frac{2 \text{ mcg}}{\text{kg min}} \left(\frac{64 \text{ kg}}{1}\right) \left(\frac{250 \text{ mL}}{4 \text{ mg}}\right) \left(\frac{1 \text{ mg}}{1000 \text{ mcg}}\right) \left(\frac{60 \text{ min}}{\text{h}}\right) = \frac{480 \text{ mL}}{\text{h}}$$

39) J.W., a 70 YO male weighing 75 kg with heart failure has an order for a continuous IV infusion of milrinone 0.6 mcg/kg/min. Milrinone is available in 100 mL bags containing 20 mg. At what rate will you set the IV infusion pump?

$$\frac{0.6 \text{ mcg}}{\text{kg min}} \left(\frac{75 \text{ kg}}{1}\right) \left(\frac{100 \text{ mL}}{20 \text{ mg}}\right) \left(\frac{1 \text{ mg}}{1000 \text{ mcg}}\right) \left(\frac{60 \text{ min}}{\text{h}}\right) = \frac{13.5 \text{ mL}}{\text{h}}$$

40) Your 55 kg 62 YO patient diagnosed with bradycardia has an order for epinephrine 0.3 mcg/kg/min IV. The efficient pharmacy sends over a bag containing 1 mg epinephrine in 250 mL NS. At what rate will you set the IV infusion pump?

$$\frac{0.3 \text{ mcg}}{\text{kg min}} \left(\frac{55 \text{ kg}}{1}\right) \left(\frac{250 \text{ mL}}{1 \text{ mg}}\right) \left(\frac{1 \text{ mg}}{1000 \text{ mcg}}\right) \left(\frac{60 \text{ min}}{\text{h}}\right) = \frac{247.5 \text{ mL}}{\text{h}}$$

Chapter 16
IV Flow Rate Adjustments

You have an order for a 500 mL bag of NS to infuse over 4 hours with a drop factor of 10. The bag was started at 1700. At 1800 you notice that 300 mL remain.

1) What is the initial calculated rate in gtts/min?

$$\frac{500 \text{ mL}}{4 \text{ h}} \left(\frac{1 \text{ h}}{60 \text{ min}}\right) \left(\frac{10 \text{ gtts}}{\text{mL}}\right) = \frac{21 \text{ gtts}}{\text{min}}$$

2) What will be the new rate in gtts/min?

$$\frac{300 \text{ mL}}{3 \text{ h}} \left(\frac{1 \text{ h}}{60 \text{ min}}\right) \left(\frac{10 \text{ gtts}}{\text{mL}}\right) = \frac{17 \text{ gtts}}{\text{min}}$$

3) What is the percent change?

$$\frac{17 - 21}{21} (100\%) = -19 \%$$

4) Will you contact the prescriber?

No

You have an order for a 1000 mL bag of NS to infuse over 3 hours with a drop factor of 15. The bag was started at 0600. At 0700 you notice that 750 mL remain.

5) What is the initial calculated rate in gtts/min?

$$\frac{1000 \text{ mL}}{3 \text{ h}} \left(\frac{1 \text{ h}}{60 \text{ min}}\right) \left(\frac{15 \text{ gtts}}{\text{mL}}\right) = \frac{83 \text{ gtts}}{\text{min}}$$

6) What will be the new rate in gtts/min?

$$\frac{750 \text{ mL}}{2 \text{ h}} \left(\frac{1 \text{ h}}{60 \text{ min}}\right) \left(\frac{15 \text{ gtts}}{\text{mL}}\right) = \frac{94 \text{ gtts}}{\text{min}}$$

7) What is the percent change?

$$\frac{94 - 83}{83} (100\%) = 13.3 \%$$

8) Will you contact the prescriber?

No

You have an order for a 1000 mL bag of D5W to infuse over 12 hours with a drop factor of 20. The bag was started at 0800. At 1400 you notice that 625 mL remain.

9) What is the initial calculated rate in gtts/min?

$$\frac{1000 \text{ mL}}{12 \text{ h}} \left(\frac{1 \text{ h}}{60 \text{ min}}\right) \left(\frac{20 \text{ gtts}}{\text{mL}}\right) = \frac{28 \text{ gtts}}{\text{min}}$$

10) What will be the new rate in gtts/min?

$$\frac{625 \text{ mL}}{6 \text{ h}} \left(\frac{1 \text{ h}}{60 \text{ min}}\right) \left(\frac{20 \text{ gtts}}{\text{mL}}\right) = \frac{35 \text{ gtts}}{\text{min}}$$

11) What is the percent change?

$$\frac{35-28}{28}(100\%) = 25\%$$

12) Will you contact the prescriber?

Yes

You have an order for a 500 mL bag of NS to infuse over 2 hours with a drop factor of 10. The bag was started at 1100. At 1130 you notice that 450 mL remain.

13) What is the initial calculated rate in gtts/min?

$$\frac{500\text{ mL}}{2\text{ h}}\left(\frac{1\text{ h}}{60\text{ min}}\right)\left(\frac{10\text{ gtts}}{\text{mL}}\right) = \frac{42\text{ gtts}}{\text{min}}$$

14) What will be the new rate in gtts/min?

$$\frac{450\text{ mL}}{1.5\text{ h}}\left(\frac{1\text{ h}}{60\text{ min}}\right)\left(\frac{10\text{ gtts}}{\text{mL}}\right) = \frac{50\text{ gtts}}{\text{min}}$$

15) What is the percent change?

$$\frac{50-42}{42}(100\%) = 19\%$$

16) Will you contact the prescriber?

No

You have an order for a 250 mL bag of NS to infuse over 2 hours with a drop factor of 60. The bag was started at 2100. At 2130 you notice that 150 mL remain.

17) What is the initial calculated rate in gtts/min?

$$\frac{250\text{ mL}}{2\text{ h}}\left(\frac{1\text{ h}}{60\text{ min}}\right)\left(\frac{60\text{ gtts}}{\text{mL}}\right) = \frac{125\text{ gtts}}{\text{min}}$$

18) What will be the new rate in gtts/min?

$$\frac{150\text{ mL}}{1.5\text{ h}}\left(\frac{1\text{ h}}{60\text{ min}}\right)\left(\frac{60\text{ gtts}}{\text{mL}}\right) = \frac{100\text{ gtts}}{\text{min}}$$

19) What is the percent change?

$$\frac{100-125}{125}(100\%) = -20\%$$

20) Will you contact the prescriber?

No

You have an order for a 1000 mL bag of D5W to infuse over 5 hours with a drop factor of 15. The bag was started at 0800. Two hours later you notice that 700 mL remain.

21) What is the initial calculated rate in gtts/min?

$$\frac{1000\text{ mL}}{5\text{ h}}\left(\frac{1\text{ h}}{60\text{ min}}\right)\left(\frac{15\text{ gtts}}{\text{mL}}\right) = \frac{50\text{ gtts}}{\text{min}}$$

22) What will be the new rate in gtts/min?

$$\frac{700 \text{ mL}}{3 \text{ h}}\left(\frac{1 \text{ h}}{60 \text{ min}}\right)\left(\frac{15 \text{ gtts}}{\text{mL}}\right) = \frac{58 \text{ gtts}}{\text{min}}$$

23) What is the percent change?

$$\frac{58-50}{50}(100\%) = 16\%$$

24) Will you contact the prescriber?

No

You have an order for a 500 mL bag of NS to infuse over 4 hours with a drop factor of 15. The bag was started at 0100. At 0300 you notice that 150 mL remain.

25) What is the initial calculated rate in gtts/min?

$$\frac{500 \text{ mL}}{4 \text{ h}}\left(\frac{1 \text{ h}}{60 \text{ min}}\right)\left(\frac{15 \text{ gtts}}{\text{mL}}\right) = \frac{31 \text{ gtts}}{\text{min}}$$

26) What will be the new rate in gtts/min?

$$\frac{150 \text{ mL}}{2 \text{ h}}\left(\frac{1 \text{ h}}{60 \text{ min}}\right)\left(\frac{15 \text{ gtts}}{\text{mL}}\right) = \frac{19 \text{ gtts}}{\text{min}}$$

27) What is the percent change?

$$\frac{19-31}{31}(100\%) = -38.7\%$$

28) Will you contact the prescriber?

Yes

You have an order for a 1000 mL bag of NS to infuse over 9 hours with a drop factor of 10. The bag was started at 1600. At 1800 you notice that 450 mL remain.

29) What is the initial calculated rate in gtts/min?

$$\frac{1000 \text{ mL}}{9 \text{ h}}\left(\frac{1 \text{ h}}{60 \text{ min}}\right)\left(\frac{10 \text{ gtts}}{\text{mL}}\right) = \frac{19 \text{ gtts}}{\text{min}}$$

30) What will be the new rate in gtts/min?

$$\frac{450 \text{ mL}}{7 \text{ h}}\left(\frac{1 \text{ h}}{60 \text{ min}}\right)\left(\frac{10 \text{ gtts}}{\text{mL}}\right) = \frac{11 \text{ gtts}}{\text{min}}$$

31) What is the percent change?

$$\frac{11-19}{19}(100\%) = -42.1\%$$

32) Will you contact the prescriber?

Yes

You have an order for a 500 mL bag of NS to infuse over 2 hours with a drop factor of 15. The bag was started at 1600. At 1700 you notice that 400 mL remain.

33) What is the initial calculated rate in gtts/min?

$$\frac{500 \text{ mL}}{2 \text{ h}}\left(\frac{1 \text{ h}}{60 \text{ min}}\right)\left(\frac{15 \text{ gtts}}{\text{mL}}\right) = \frac{63 \text{ gtts}}{\text{min}}$$

34) What will be the new rate in gtts/min?

$$\frac{400 \text{ mL}}{\text{h}}\left(\frac{1 \text{ h}}{60 \text{ min}}\right)\left(\frac{15 \text{ gtts}}{\text{mL}}\right) = \frac{100 \text{ gtts}}{\text{min}}$$

35) What is the percent change?

$$\frac{100 - 63}{63}(100\%) = 58.7\,\%$$

36) Will you contact the prescriber?

Yes

You have an order for a 500 mL bag of NS to infuse over 7 hours with a drop factor of 20. The bag was started at 1900. At 2000 you notice that 300 mL remain.

37) What is the initial calculated rate in gtts/min?

$$\frac{500 \text{ mL}}{7 \text{ h}}\left(\frac{1 \text{ h}}{60 \text{ min}}\right)\left(\frac{20 \text{ gtts}}{\text{mL}}\right) = \frac{24 \text{ gtts}}{\text{min}}$$

38) What will be the new rate in gtts/min?

$$\frac{300 \text{ mL}}{6 \text{ h}}\left(\frac{1 \text{ h}}{60 \text{ min}}\right)\left(\frac{20 \text{ gtts}}{\text{mL}}\right) = \frac{17 \text{ gtts}}{\text{min}}$$

39) What is the percent change?

$$\frac{17 - 24}{24}(100\%) = -29.2\,\%$$

40) Will you contact the prescriber?

Yes

Chapter 17
Heparin Infusion and Adjustment Calculations

Pt A.K., who weighs 190 lb, has been admitted with a diagnosis of DVT and has the following heparin order:
Initial bolus: 80 units/kg (max 10,000 units)
Initial infusion: 18 units/kg/h (initial max of 1800 units/h)
1) Calculate the bolus dose in units.

$$\frac{80 \text{ units}}{\text{kg}} \left(\frac{190 \text{ lb}}{1}\right)\left(\frac{1 \text{ kg}}{2.2 \text{ lb}}\right) = 6909 \text{ units rounded to } 7000 \text{ units}$$

2) Calculate the bolus dose in mL.

$$7000 \text{ units}\left(\frac{1 \text{ mL}}{5000 \text{ units}}\right) = 1.4 \text{ mL}$$

3) Calculate the initial infusion rate in units/h.

$$\frac{18 \text{ units}}{\text{kg h}}\left(\frac{190 \text{ lb}}{1}\right)\left(\frac{1 \text{ kg}}{2.2 \text{ lb}}\right) = \frac{1555 \text{ units}}{\text{h}} \text{ rounded to } \frac{1600 \text{ units}}{\text{h}}$$

4) Calculate the initial infusion rate in mL/h.

$$\frac{1600 \text{ units}}{\text{h}}\left(\frac{1 \text{ mL}}{100 \text{ units}}\right) = \frac{16 \text{ mL}}{\text{h}}$$

5) The initial infusion was started at 1300. At 1900 you order an anti-Xa assay and it comes back at 0.75 units/mL. What will the new infusion rate be in units/h?

Decrease by 1 unit/kg/h resulting in new rate of 17 units/kg/h.

$$\frac{17 \text{ units}}{\text{kg h}}\left(\frac{190 \text{ lb}}{1}\right)\left(\frac{1 \text{ kg}}{2.2 \text{ lb}}\right) = \frac{1468 \text{ units}}{\text{h}} \text{ rounded to } \frac{1500 \text{ units}}{\text{h}}$$

6) At 0100 the following day another anti-Xa assay is ordered and comes back at 0.69 units/mL. Will you, or the on-duty nurse, adjust the dose? If so, what will the new infusion rate be in units/h?

No dosage adjustment.

7) At 0700 another anti-Xa assay is ordered which comes back at 0.70 units/mL. What do you do?

No dosage adjustment and decrease to daily monitoring.

Pt B.J., who weighs 194 lb, has been admitted with a diagnosis of unstable angina and has the following heparin order:
Initial bolus: 60 units/kg (max 5,000 units)
Initial infusion: 12 units/kg/h (initial max of 1000 units/h)
8) Calculate the bolus dose in units.

$$\frac{60 \text{ units}}{\text{kg}}\left(\frac{194 \text{ lb}}{1}\right)\left(\frac{1 \text{ kg}}{2.2 \text{ lb}}\right) = 5291 \text{ units which exceeds maximum of } 5000 \text{ units}$$

Initial bolus is 5000 units.

9) Calculate the bolus dose in mL.

$$5000 \text{ units} \left(\frac{1 \text{ mL}}{5000 \text{ units}}\right) = 1 \text{ mL}$$

10) Calculate the initial infusion rate in units/h.

$$\frac{12 \text{ units}}{\text{kg h}} \left(\frac{194 \text{ lb}}{1}\right)\left(\frac{1 \text{ kg}}{2.2 \text{ lb}}\right) = \frac{1058 \text{ units}}{\text{h}} \text{ which exceeds maximum of } \frac{1000 \text{ units}}{\text{h}}$$

Initial infusion rate is 1000 units/h.

11) Calculate the initial infusion rate in mL/h.

$$\frac{1000 \text{ units}}{\text{h}} \left(\frac{1 \text{ mL}}{100 \text{ units}}\right) = \frac{10 \text{ mL}}{\text{h}}$$

12) The initial infusion was started at 1400. At 2000 you order an anti-Xa assay and it comes back at 0.25 units/mL. What course of action will you take? Include all calculations.

Re-bolus at 40 units/kg.

$$\frac{40 \text{ units}}{\text{kg}} \left(\frac{194 \text{ lb}}{1}\right)\left(\frac{1 \text{ kg}}{2.2 \text{ lb}}\right) = 3527 \text{ units rounded to 3500 units}$$

$$3500 \text{ units} \left(\frac{1 \text{ mL}}{5000 \text{ units}}\right) = 0.7 \text{ mL}$$

Increase infusion by 2 units/kg/h resulting in new rate of 14 units/kg/h.

$$\frac{14 \text{ units}}{\text{kg h}} \left(\frac{194 \text{ lb}}{1}\right)\left(\frac{1 \text{ kg}}{2.2 \text{ lb}}\right) = \frac{1234 \text{ units}}{\text{h}} \text{ rounded to } \frac{1200 \text{ units}}{\text{h}}$$

$$\frac{1200 \text{ units}}{\text{h}} \left(\frac{1 \text{ mL}}{100 \text{ units}}\right) = \frac{12 \text{ mL}}{\text{h}}$$

13) At 0200 the following day another anti-Xa assay is ordered and comes back at 0.51 units/mL. Will you, or the on-duty nurse, adjust the dose? If so, what will the new infusion rate be in units/h?

No dosage adjustment.

14) At 0800 another anti-Xa assay is ordered which comes back at 0.72 units/mL. What do you do?

Decrease dosage by 1 unit/kg/h resulting in new rate of 13 units/kg/h.

$$\frac{13 \text{ units}}{\text{kg h}} \left(\frac{194 \text{ lb}}{1}\right)\left(\frac{1 \text{ kg}}{2.2 \text{ lb}}\right) = \frac{1146 \text{ units}}{\text{h}} \text{ rounded to } \frac{1100 \text{ units}}{\text{h}}$$

$$\frac{1100 \text{ units}}{\text{h}} \left(\frac{1 \text{ mL}}{100 \text{ units}}\right) = \frac{11 \text{ mL}}{\text{h}}$$

Pt A.R., a 45 YO female weighing 135 lb, has been admitted with a diagnosis of PE and has the following heparin order:
Initial bolus: 80 units/kg (max 10,000 units)
Initial infusion: 18 units/kg/h (initial max of 1800 units/h)

15) Calculate the bolus dose in units.

$$\frac{80 \text{ units}}{\text{kg}} \left(\frac{135 \text{ lb}}{1}\right)\left(\frac{1 \text{ kg}}{2.2 \text{ lb}}\right) = 4909 \text{ units rounded to 5000 units}$$

16) Calculate the bolus dose in mL.

$$5000 \text{ units} \left(\frac{1 \text{ mL}}{5000 \text{ units}}\right) = 1 \text{ mL}$$

17) Calculate the initial infusion rate in units/h.

$$\frac{18 \text{ units}}{\text{kg h}} \left(\frac{135 \text{ lb}}{1}\right)\left(\frac{1 \text{ kg}}{2.2 \text{ lb}}\right) = \frac{1105 \text{ units}}{\text{h}} \text{ rounded to } \frac{1100 \text{ units}}{\text{h}}$$

18) Calculate the initial infusion rate in mL/h.

$$\frac{1100 \text{ units}}{\text{h}} \left(\frac{1 \text{ mL}}{100 \text{ units}}\right) = \frac{11 \text{ mL}}{\text{h}}$$

19) The initial infusion was started at 0930. At 3:30 PM you order an anti-Xa assay and it comes back at 0.95 units/mL. What course of action will you take? What will the new infusion rate be in units/h?

Hold infusion for 60 minutes.

Decrease dosage by 3 units/kg/h resulting in new rate of 15 units/kg/h.

$$\frac{15 \text{ units}}{\text{kg h}} \left(\frac{135 \text{ lb}}{1}\right)\left(\frac{1 \text{ kg}}{2.2 \text{ lb}}\right) = \frac{920 \text{ units}}{\text{h}} \text{ rounded to } \frac{900 \text{ units}}{\text{h}}$$

20) At 2130 another anti-Xa assay is ordered and comes back at 0.91 units/mL. What is your course of action?

Two consecutive anti-Xa assays have come back > 0.9. Contact prescriber for course of action.

21) After contacting the prescriber after the second anti-Xa assay >9.0, you are instructed to hold the infusion for 60 minutes and decrease the dosage by 3 units/kg/h. What will be the new rate in units/h?

$$\frac{12 \text{ units}}{\text{kg h}} \left(\frac{135 \text{ lb}}{1}\right)\left(\frac{1 \text{ kg}}{2.2 \text{ lb}}\right) = \frac{736 \text{ units}}{\text{h}} \text{ rounded to } \frac{700 \text{ units}}{\text{h}}$$

Pt J.W., who weighs 74 kg, has been admitted with a diagnosis of stroke and has the following heparin order:
Initial bolus: None
Initial infusion: 12 units/kg/h (initial max of 1200 units/h)
22) Calculate the bolus dose in units.

No bolus is given.

23) Calculate the bolus dose in mL.

No bolus is given.

24) Calculate the initial infusion rate in units/h.

$$\frac{12 \text{ units}}{\text{kg h}} \left(\frac{74 \text{ kg}}{1}\right) = \frac{888 \text{ units}}{\text{h}} \text{ rounded to } \frac{900 \text{ units}}{\text{h}}$$

25) Calculate the initial infusion rate in mL/h.

$$\frac{900 \text{ units}}{\text{h}} \left(\frac{1 \text{ mL}}{100 \text{ units}}\right) = \frac{9 \text{ mL}}{\text{h}}$$

26) The initial infusion was started at 6:30 AM. At 12:30 PM you order an anti-Xa assay and it comes back at 0.53 units/mL. What will the new infusion rate be in units/h?

No dosage adjustment.

27) At 6:30 PM another anti-Xa assay is ordered and comes back at 0.51 units/mL. Will you, or the on-duty nurse, adjust the dose? If so, what will the new infusion rate be in mL/h?

No dosage adjustment.

28) At 0700 another anti-Xa assay is ordered which comes back at 0.53 units/mL. What do you do? When will you order the next anti-Xa?

No dosage adjustment. Next anti-Xa assay is at 0700 the next day.

Pt T.G, who weighs 86 kg, has been admitted with a diagnosis of DVT and has the following heparin order:
Initial bolus: 80 units/kg (max 10,000 units)
Initial infusion: 18 units/kg/h (initial max of 1800 units/h)

29) Calculate the bolus dose in units.

$$\frac{80 \text{ units}}{\text{kg}} \left(\frac{86 \text{ kg}}{1}\right) = 6880 \text{ units rounded to } 7000 \text{ units}$$

30) Calculate the bolus dose in mL.

$$7000 \text{ units} \left(\frac{1 \text{ mL}}{5000 \text{ units}}\right) = 1.4 \text{ mL}$$

31) Calculate the initial infusion rate in units/h.

$$\frac{18 \text{ units}}{\text{kg h}} \left(\frac{86 \text{ kg}}{1}\right) = \frac{1548 \text{ units}}{\text{h}} \text{ rounded to } \frac{1500 \text{ units}}{\text{h}}$$

32) Calculate the initial infusion rate in mL/h.

$$\frac{1500 \text{ units}}{\text{h}} \left(\frac{1 \text{ mL}}{100 \text{ units}}\right) = \frac{15 \text{ mL}}{\text{h}}$$

33) The initial infusion was started at 1300. At 1900 you order an anti-Xa assay and it comes back at 0.75 units/mL. What will the new infusion rate be in units/h?

Decrease dosage by 1 unit/kg/h resulting in new rate of 17 units/kg/h.

$$\frac{17 \text{ units}}{\text{kg h}} \left(\frac{86 \text{ kg}}{1}\right) = \frac{1462 \text{ units}}{\text{h}} \text{ rounded to } \frac{1500 \text{ units}}{\text{h}}$$

The rate remains constant at 1500 units/h due to rounding rules. Check anti-Xa level again in 6 hours.

34) At 0100 the following day another anti-Xa assay is ordered and comes back at 0.69 units/mL. Will you, or the on-duty nurse, adjust the dose? If so, what will the new infusion rate be in units/h?

No dosage adjustment.

35) At 0700 another anti-Xa assay is ordered which comes back at 0.70 units/mL. What do you do?

No dosage adjustment. Two consecutive anti-Xa levels are within therapeutic range, so decrease to daily monitoring.

Pt M.J., who weighs 109 kg, has been admitted with a diagnosis of DVT and has the following heparin order:
Initial bolus: 80 units/kg (max 10,000 units)
Initial infusion: 18 units/kg/h (initial max of 1800 units/h)

36) Calculate the bolus dose in units.

$$\frac{80 \text{ units}}{\text{kg}} \left(\frac{109 \text{ kg}}{1}\right) = 8720 \text{ units rounded to } 8500 \text{ units}$$

37) Calculate the bolus dose in mL.

$$8500 \text{ units} \left(\frac{1 \text{ mL}}{5000 \text{ units}}\right) = 1.7 \text{ mL}$$

38) Calculate the initial infusion rate in units/h.

$$\frac{18 \text{ units}}{\text{kg h}} \left(\frac{109 \text{ kg}}{1}\right) = \frac{1962 \text{ units}}{\text{h}} \text{ which exceeds maximum of } \frac{1800 \text{ units}}{\text{h}}$$

Initial infusion rate is 1800 units/h.

39) Calculate the initial infusion rate in mL/h.

$$\frac{1800 \text{ units}}{\text{h}} \left(\frac{1 \text{ mL}}{100 \text{ units}}\right) = \frac{18 \text{ mL}}{\text{h}}$$

40) The initial infusion was started at 1015. At 1615 you order an anti-Xa assay and it comes back at 0.24 units/mL. What is your course of action? Show all calculations.

Re-bolus at 40 units/kg.

$$\frac{40 \text{ units}}{\text{kg}} \left(\frac{109 \text{ kg}}{1}\right) = 4360 \text{ units rounded to } 4500 \text{ units}$$

$$4500 \text{ units} \left(\frac{1 \text{ mL}}{5000 \text{ units}}\right) = 0.9 \text{ mL}$$

Increase infusion by 2 units/kg/h resulting in new rate of 20 units/kg/h.

$$\frac{20 \text{ units}}{\text{kg h}} \left(\frac{109 \text{ kg}}{1}\right) = \frac{2180 \text{ units}}{\text{h}} \text{ rounded to } \frac{2200 \text{ units}}{\text{h}}$$

$$\frac{2200 \text{ units}}{\text{h}} \left(\frac{1 \text{ mL}}{100 \text{ units}}\right) = \frac{22 \text{ mL}}{\text{h}}$$

41) At 2215 another anti-Xa assay is ordered and comes back at 0.41 units/mL. Will you, or the on-duty nurse, adjust the dose? If so, what will the new infusion rate be in units/h?

No dosage adjustment.

42) At 0415 another anti-Xa assay is ordered which comes back at 0.45 units/mL. What do you do?

No dosage adjustment. Two consecutive anti-Xa levels are within therapeutic range, so decrease to daily monitoring.

Pt T.W., who weighs 69 kg, has been admitted with a diagnosis of DVT and has the following heparin order:
Initial bolus: 80 units/kg (max 10,000 units)
Initial infusion: 18 units/kg/h (initial max of 1800 units/h)
43) Calculate the bolus dose in units.

$$\frac{80 \text{ units}}{\text{kg}} \left(\frac{69 \text{ kg}}{1}\right) = 5520 \text{ units rounded to } 5500 \text{ units}$$

44) Calculate the bolus dose in mL.

$$5500 \text{ units} \left(\frac{1 \text{ mL}}{5000 \text{ units}}\right) = 1.1 \text{ mL}$$

45) Calculate the initial infusion rate in units/h.

$$\frac{18 \text{ units}}{\text{kg h}} \left(\frac{69 \text{ kg}}{1}\right) = \frac{1242 \text{ units}}{\text{h}} \text{ rounded to } \frac{1200 \text{ units}}{\text{h}}$$

46) Calculate the initial infusion rate in mL/h.

$$\frac{1200 \text{ units}}{h}\left(\frac{1 \text{ mL}}{100 \text{ units}}\right) = \frac{12 \text{ mL}}{h}$$

47) The initial infusion was started at 0600. At 1200 you order an anti-Xa assay and it comes back at 0.82 units/mL. What is your course of action? What will the new infusion rate be in units/h?

Hold infusion for 30 minutes.

Decrease dosage by 2 units/kg/h resulting in new rate of 16 units/kg/h.

$$\frac{16 \text{ units}}{\text{kg h}}\left(\frac{69 \text{ kg}}{1}\right) = \frac{1104 \text{ units}}{h} \text{ rounded to } \frac{1100 \text{ units}}{h}$$

48) At 1800 another anti-Xa assay is ordered and comes back at 0.74 units/mL. Will you, or the on-duty nurse, adjust the dose? If so, what will the new infusion rate be in units/h?

Decrease dosage by 1 unit/kg/h resulting in new rate of 15 units/kg/h.

$$\frac{15 \text{ units}}{\text{kg h}}\left(\frac{69 \text{ kg}}{1}\right) = \frac{1035 \text{ units}}{h} \text{ rounded to } \frac{1000 \text{ units}}{h}$$

49) At 0000 another anti-Xa assay is ordered which comes back at 0.71 units/mL. What do you do? If you adjust the dosage, what is the new rate in mL/h?

Decrease dosage by 1 unit/kg/h resulting in new rate of 14 units/kg/h.

$$\frac{14 \text{ units}}{\text{kg h}}\left(\frac{69 \text{ kg}}{1}\right) = \frac{966 \text{ units}}{h} \text{ rounded to } \frac{1000 \text{ units}}{h}$$

The rate remains constant at 1000 units/h due to rounding rules. Check anti-Xa level again in 6 hours.

Pt W.W., who weighs 46 kg, has been admitted with a diagnosis of PE and has the following heparin order:
Initial bolus: 80 units/kg (max 10,000 units)
Initial infusion: 18 units/kg/h (initial max of 1800 units/h)

50) Calculate the bolus dose in units.

$$\frac{80 \text{ units}}{\text{kg}}\left(\frac{46 \text{ kg}}{1}\right) = 3680 \text{ units rounded to } 3500 \text{ units}$$

51) Calculate the bolus dose in mL.

$$3500 \text{ units}\left(\frac{1 \text{ mL}}{5000 \text{ units}}\right) = 0.7 \text{ mL}$$

52) Calculate the initial infusion rate in units/h.

$$\frac{18 \text{ units}}{\text{kg h}}\left(\frac{46 \text{ kg}}{1}\right) = \frac{828 \text{ units}}{h} \text{ rounded to } \frac{800 \text{ units}}{h}$$

53) Calculate the initial infusion rate in mL/h.

$$\frac{800 \text{ units}}{h}\left(\frac{1 \text{ mL}}{100 \text{ units}}\right) = \frac{8 \text{ mL}}{h}$$

54) The initial infusion was started at 1100. At 1700 you order an anti-Xa assay and it comes back at 0.22 units/mL. What course of action do you take? Show calculations.

Re-bolus at 40 units/kg.

$$\frac{40 \text{ units}}{\text{kg}}\left(\frac{46 \text{ kg}}{1}\right) = 1840 \text{ units rounded to } 2000 \text{ units}$$

$$2000 \text{ units}\left(\frac{1 \text{ mL}}{5000 \text{ units}}\right) = 0.4 \text{ mL}$$

Increase infusion by 2 units/kg/h resulting in new rate of 20 units/kg/h.

$$\frac{20 \text{ units}}{\text{kg h}}\left(\frac{46 \text{ kg}}{1}\right) = \frac{920 \text{ units}}{\text{h}} \text{ rounded to } \frac{900 \text{ units}}{\text{h}}$$

$$\frac{900 \text{ units}}{\text{h}}\left(\frac{1 \text{ mL}}{100 \text{ units}}\right) = \frac{9 \text{ mL}}{\text{h}}$$

55) At 2300 another anti-Xa assay is ordered and comes back at 0.40 units/mL. Will you, or the on-duty nurse, adjust the dose? If so, what will the new infusion rate be in units/h?

No dosage adjustment.

56) At 0500 the next day, another anti-Xa assay is ordered which comes back at 0.42 units/mL. What do you do?

No dosage adjustment. Two consecutive anti-Xa levels are within therapeutic range, so decrease to daily monitoring.

Pt J.J., a 72 YO male weighing 85 kg has been admitted with a diagnosis of unstable angina and has the following heparin order:
Initial bolus: 60 units/kg (max 5,000 units)
Initial infusion: 12 units/kg/h (initial max of 1000 units/h)

57) Calculate the bolus dose in units.

$$\frac{60 \text{ units}}{\text{kg}}\left(\frac{85 \text{ kg}}{1}\right) = 5100 \text{ units rounded to } 5000 \text{ units}$$

58) Calculate the bolus dose in mL.

$$5000 \text{ units}\left(\frac{1 \text{ mL}}{5000 \text{ units}}\right) = 1 \text{ mL}$$

59) Calculate the initial infusion rate in units/h.

$$\frac{12 \text{ units}}{\text{kg h}}\left(\frac{85 \text{ kg}}{1}\right) = \frac{1020 \text{ units}}{\text{h}} \text{ rounded to } \frac{1000 \text{ units}}{\text{h}}$$

60) Calculate the initial infusion rate in mL/h.

$$\frac{1000 \text{ units}}{\text{h}}\left(\frac{1 \text{ mL}}{100 \text{ units}}\right) = \frac{10 \text{ mL}}{\text{h}}$$

61) The initial infusion was started at 1600. At 2200 you order an anti-Xa assay and it comes back at 0.82 units/mL. What course of action will you take? Include all calculations.

Hold infusion for 30 minutes.

Decrease dosage by 2 units/kg/h resulting in new rate of 10 units/kg/h.

$$\frac{10 \text{ units}}{\text{kg h}} \left(\frac{85 \text{ kg}}{1}\right) = \frac{850 \text{ units}}{\text{h}} \text{ rounded to } \frac{900 \text{ units}}{\text{h}}$$

$$\frac{900 \text{ units}}{\text{h}} \left(\frac{1 \text{ mL}}{100 \text{ units}}\right) = \frac{9 \text{ mL}}{\text{h}}$$

62) At 0400 the following day another anti-Xa assay is ordered and comes back at 0.75 units/mL. Will you, or the on-duty nurse, adjust the dose? If so, what will the new infusion rate be in units/h?

Yes, decrease dosage by 1 unit/kg/h resulting in new rate of 9 units/kg/h.

$$\frac{9 \text{ units}}{\text{kg h}} \left(\frac{85 \text{ kg}}{1}\right) = \frac{765 \text{ units}}{\text{h}} \text{ rounded to } \frac{800 \text{ units}}{\text{h}}$$

63) At 1000 another anti-Xa assay is ordered which comes back at 0.71 units/mL. What do you do?

Decrease dosage by 1 unit/kg/h resulting in new rate of 8 units/kg/h.

$$\frac{8 \text{ units}}{\text{kg h}} \left(\frac{85 \text{ kg}}{1}\right) = \frac{680 \text{ units}}{\text{h}} \text{ rounded to } \frac{700 \text{ units}}{\text{h}}$$

Chapter 18
Percent

Convert the following numbers to percents.

Problem	Number	Percent
Example	0.37	0.37 (100%) = 37%
1	0.21	0.21 (100%) = 21%
2	0.88	0.88 (100%) = 88%
3	2.38	02.38 (100%) = 238%
4	3.89	3.89 (100%) = 389%
5	0.005	0.005 (100%) = 0.5%
6	0.02	0.02 (100%) = 2%
7	1.35	1.35 (100%) = 135%
8	0.41	0.41 (100%) = 41%
9	0.69	0.69 (100%) = 69%
10	7.55	7.55 (100%) = 755%

Convert the following percents to numbers.

Problem	Percent	Number
Example	32%	32%/100% = 0.32
11	42.5%	42.5%/100% = 0.425
12	89%	89%/100% = 0.89
13	1.1%	1.1%/100% = 0.011
14	64.3%	64.3%/100% = 0.643
15	5.6%	5.6%/100% = 0.056
16	4.35%	4.35%/100% = 0.0435
17	3.9%	3.9%/100% = 0.039
18	5.2%	5.2%/100% = 0.052
19	1.7%	1.7%/100% = 0.017
20	0.3%	0.3%/100% = 0.003

Chapter 19
Percent Strength

Express the following as percent strength solutions and include the type of solution (w/w, w/v, v/v, v/w).

1) 2.45 g NaCl in 2 L

(2.45 g/2L) (1 L/1000 mL) 100%= 0.12% w/v

2) 1 g HC in 200 g HC ointment

(1 g AI/200 g) 100% = 0.5% w/w

3) 10 g urea in 40 g urea ointment

(10 g AI/40 g) 100% = 25% w/w

4) 20 mL ETOH in 100 mL ETOH solution

(20 mL ETOH/100 mL) 100% = 20% v/v

5) 2.5 mg betamethasone in 10 g betamethasone ointment

(2.5 mg AI/10 g) (1 g AI/1000 mg AI) 100% = 0.025% w/w

6) 25 mcg NaCl in 0.25 mL

(25 mcg /0.25 mL) (1 g /1,000,000 mcg) 100% = 0.01% w/v

7) 510 mg NaHCO$_3$ in 200 mL

(510 mg/200 mL) (1 g/1000 mg) 100% = 0.255% w/v

8) 7.5 g NaCl in 1000 mL

(7.5 g/1000 mL) 100% = 0.75% w/v

9) 5 g KCl in 200 mL

(5 g/200 mL) 100% = 2.5% w/v

10) 10 g salicylic acid in 200 g salicylic acid cream

(10 g AI/200 g)100% = 5% w/w

Answer the following:

11) How many mg of bupivacaine are in 45 mL of 0.5% bupivacaine solution?

$$45 \text{ mL} \left(\frac{0.5 \text{ g}}{100 \text{ mL}}\right)\left(\frac{1000 \text{ mg}}{\text{g}}\right) = 225 \text{ mg}$$

12) How many mg of NaCl are in 60 mL of 0.9% NaCl (normal saline)?

$$60 \text{ mL} \left(\frac{0.9 \text{ g}}{100 \text{ mL}}\right)\left(\frac{1000 \text{ mg}}{\text{g}}\right) = 540 \text{ mg}$$

13) How many mg of lidocaine are in 250 mL of 1% lidocaine?

$$250 \text{ mL} \left(\frac{1 \text{ g}}{100 \text{ mL}}\right)\left(\frac{1000 \text{ mg}}{\text{g}}\right) = 2500 \text{ mg}$$

14) How many g of KCl are in 473 mL of 10% KCl?

$$473 \text{ mL} \left(\frac{10 \text{ g}}{100 \text{ mL}}\right) = 47.3 \text{ g}$$

15) How many mcg of dextrose are in 1 drop of 5% dextrose solution if there are 20 drops/mL?

$$1 \text{ gtt} \left(\frac{1 \text{ mL}}{20 \text{ gtts}}\right) \left(\frac{5 \text{ g}}{100 \text{ mL}}\right) \left(\frac{1,000,000 \text{ mcg}}{\text{g}}\right) = 2500 \text{ mcg}$$

16) How many g of NaCl are in 1.5 L of NS (normal saline-0.9% NaCl)?

$$1.5 \text{ L} \left(\frac{1000 \text{ mL}}{\text{L}}\right) \left(\frac{0.9 \text{ g}}{100 \text{ mL}}\right) = 13.5 \text{ g}$$

17) How many mg of triamcinolone are in 60 g of 0.1% triamcinolone ointment?

$$60 \text{ g} \left(\frac{0.1 \text{ g AI}}{100 \text{ g}}\right) \left(\frac{1000 \text{ mg AI}}{\text{g AI}}\right) = 60 \text{ mg AI}$$

18) How many g of HC are in 200 g of 2.5% HC ointment?

$$200 \text{ g} \left(\frac{2.5 \text{ g AI}}{100 \text{ g}}\right) = 5 \text{ g AI}$$

19) How many mcg of fluocinolone are in 50 g of 0.01% fluocinolone cream?

$$50 \text{ g} \left(\frac{0.01 \text{ g AI}}{100 \text{ g}}\right) \left(\frac{1,000,000 \text{ mcg AI}}{\text{g AI}}\right) = 5000 \text{ mcg AI}$$

20) How many grams of dextrose are in 2 L of D5W (5% dextrose in water)?

$$2 \text{ L} \left(\frac{1000 \text{ mL}}{\text{L}}\right) \left(\frac{5 \text{ g}}{100 \text{ mL}}\right) = 100 \text{ g}$$

Chapter 20
Percent Change

- The formula to calculate percent change is:

$$\frac{\text{Final} - \text{Initial}}{\text{Initial}} (100\%) = \%\text{ Change}$$

- Remember, the percent change can be positive or negative.
- If the units are the same, they will cancel out and there is no need to include them in the calculations.

Calculate the percent change in the following scenarios. Round to the nearest tenth percent.

1) Your patient weighed 86 kg on admission and weighs 82 kg today.

((82-86)/86) 100% = -4.7%

2) Your patient weighed 194 lb on admission and weighs 197 lb today.

((197-194)/194) 100% = 1.5%

3) A patient's daily dose of a drug was reduced from 45 mg to 40 mg.

((40-45)/45) 100% = -11.1%

4) The number of patients in your unit increased from 9 to 12.

((12-9)/9) 100% = 33.3%

5) You increase an IV flow rate from 6.5 mL/h to 8 mL/h.

((8-6.5)/6.5) 100% = 23.1%

6) The number of tacos in the breakroom decreased from 12 to 5.

((5-12)/12) 100% = -58.3%

7) You got a merit raise from $47.45/h to $49.05/h.

((49.05-47.45)/47.45) 100% = 3.4%

8) Your patient, who you encouraged to exercise and watch his diet, weighed 205 lb one month ago and now weighs 195 lb.

((195-205)/205) 100% = -4.9%

9) A dosage increased from 10 mg b.i.d to 20 mg b.i.d.

((20-10)/10) 100% = 100%

10) A patient weighed 78 kg on Monday and still weighs 78 kg on Thursday.

((78-78)/78) 100% = 0%

11) You had to adjust an IV drip from 32 gtt/min to 38 gtt/min.

((38-32)/32) 100% = 18.8%

12) You start a diet and reduce your caloric intake from 4500 kcal/day to 2500 kcal/day.

((2500-4500)/4500) 100% = -44.4%

13) You can now do 25 pushups but a month ago you could only do 10.

((25-10)/10) 100% = 150%

14) You have a spouse and two kids on Monday. On Tuesday you have triplets. What is the percent change in total family members?

((7-4)/4) 100% = 75%

15) You own 7 cats and go to the shelter and adopt 2 more cats.

((9-7)/7) 100% = 28.6%

16) You ran a marathon in 6 hours in 2016. In 2019 you run the same marathon in 5 hours.

((5-6)/6) 100% = -16.7%

17) The distance you drive to work is 8.0 miles. On Monday you average 40 mph and it takes you 12 minutes. On Tuesday you average 80 mph and it takes you 6 minutes.

a) Calculate percent change in speed.

((80-40)/40) 100% = 100%

b) Calculate the percent change in time of commute.

((6-12)/12) 100% = -50%

c) Calculate the percent change in distance traveled.

((8-8)/8) 100% = 0%

18) Your patient's serum potassium level decreased from 4.1 mEq/L to 3.9 mEq/L.

((3.9-4.1)/4.1) 100% = -4.9%

19) One of your nine cats leaves you to live with the neighbor (better food, more petting).

((8-9)/9) 100% = -11.1%

20) You watched your diet and exercised, and your LDL decreased from 130 mg/dL to 120 mg/dL.

((120-130)/130) 100% = -7.7%

21) You increased a Pitocin drip from 2 milliunits/minute to 3 milliunits/minute.

((3-2)/2) 100% = 50%

22) A patient had his atorvastatin dosage lowered from 80 mg once daily to 40 mg once daily.

((40-80)/80) 100% = -50%

23) You notice the 99 Cent Store raised the price of dental floss from 99 cents to 99.9 cents.

((99.9-99)/99) 100% = 0.9%

24) You turned 30 today. What percent change have you aged in the last year?

((30-29)/29) 100% = 3.4%

25) The physician reduced a patient's daily dose from 10 mg to zero.

((0-10)/10) 100% = -100%

Chapter 21
Ratio Strength

1) How many mg of active ingredient are in 400 mL of a 1:10,000 solution?

$$400 \text{ mL} \left(\frac{1 \text{ g}}{10,000 \text{ mL}}\right)\left(\frac{1000 \text{ mg}}{\text{g}}\right) = 40 \text{ mg}$$

2) How many mcg are in 100 mL of a 1:100,000 solution?

$$100 \text{ mL} \left(\frac{1 \text{ g}}{100,000 \text{ mL}}\right)\left(\frac{1,000,000 \text{ mcg}}{\text{g}}\right) = 1000 \text{ mcg}$$

3) You have a 10 mL vial which is labeled 1:10,000 and are asked to draw up 0.5 mg of drug. How many mL would you draw?

$$0.5 \text{ mg} \left(\frac{10,000 \text{ mL}}{\text{g}}\right)\left(\frac{1 \text{ g}}{1000 \text{ mg}}\right) = 5 \text{ mL}$$

4) How many grams of active ingredient are in 60 mL of a 1:200 solution?

$$60 \text{ mL} \left(\frac{1 \text{ g}}{200 \text{ mL}}\right) = 0.3 \text{ g}$$

5) How many grams of active ingredient are in 500 g of a 1:50 w/w preparation?

$$500 \text{ g} \left(\frac{1 \text{ g AI}}{50 \text{ g}}\right) = 10 \text{ g AI}$$

6) You have a 50 mL vial which is labeled 1:1000 and are asked to draw up 1.2 mg. How many mL would you draw?

$$1.2 \text{ mg} \left(\frac{1000 \text{ mL}}{1 \text{ g}}\right)\left(\frac{1 \text{ g}}{1000 \text{ mg}}\right) = 1.2 \text{ mL}$$

7) You have a solution which is 1:1000 w/v. What is the percent strength?

$$\left(\frac{1 \text{ g}}{1000 \text{ mL}}\right) 100\% = 0.1\%$$

8) What is the percent strength of a 1:100 w/v solution?

$$\left(\frac{1 \text{ g}}{100 \text{ mL}}\right) 100\% = 1\%$$

9) How many grams of active ingredient are in 100 mL of a 1:10,000 solution?

$$100 \text{ mL} \left(\frac{1 \text{ g}}{10,000 \text{ mL}}\right) = 0.01 \text{ g}$$

10) You have a 100 mL vial which is labeled 1:1000. How many mg are in 50 mL of the solution?

$$50 \text{ mL} \left(\frac{1 \text{ g}}{1000 \text{ mL}}\right)\left(\frac{1000 \text{ mg}}{\text{g}}\right) = 50 \text{ mg}$$

Chapter 22
Reconstitution Calculations

1) A 1 g vial states to add 8.1 mL of SW for injection for a final concentration of 100 mg/mL. You have an order for 250 mg IV. How many mL will you administer?

$$250 \text{ mg}\left(\frac{1 \text{ mL}}{100 \text{ mg}}\right) = 2.5 \text{ mL}$$

2) The physician has ordered 300 mg IM of a drug which is available in a 1000 mg vial with directions to add 4.6 mL SW for injection for a final concentration of 200 mg/mL. How many mL will you administer?

$$300 \text{ mg}\left(\frac{1 \text{ mL}}{200 \text{ mg}}\right) = 1.5 \text{ mL}$$

3) You have an order for 400 mg IM of a drug which is available in 1 g vials with directions to reconstitute with 8.5 mL of SW for injection for a final concentration of 100 mg/mL. How many mL will you administer?

$$400 \text{ mg}\left(\frac{1 \text{ mL}}{100 \text{ mg}}\right) = 4 \text{ mL}$$

4) A 1,000,000-unit vial of penicillin G potassium has instructions which state to reconstitute to a concentration of 100,000 units per mL, add 10 mL SW for injection. You have an order for 200,000 units IM. How many mL will you administer?

$$200,000 \text{ units}\left(\frac{1 \text{ mL}}{100,000 \text{ units}}\right) = 2 \text{ mL}$$

5) A 65 kg male patient diagnosed with herpes simplex encephalitis is to receive acyclovir 10 mg/kg IV infused over 1 hour, every 8 hours for 10 days. You have on hand a 1000 mg vial with the instructions to dissolve the contents of the vial in 20 mL of SWFI with the resulting solution containing 50 mg of acyclovir per mL. The calculated dose will then be withdrawn and added to a 100 mL bag of D5W. After reconstitution, what volume of the 50 mg/mL solution will you add to the 100 mL bag?

$$65 \text{ kg}\left(\frac{10 \text{ mg}}{\text{kg}}\right)\left(\frac{1 \text{ mL}}{50 \text{ mg}}\right) = 13 \text{ mL}$$

6) You are reconstituting a 150 mL bottle of amoxicillin 250 mg/5 mL. The instructions for reconstitution are as follows. Total amount of water required for reconstitution is 111 mL. Tap the bottle until all powder flows freely. Add approximately 1/3 of the total amount of water for reconstitution and shake vigorously to wet the powder. Add the remainder of the water and again shake vigorously. How long would the bottle last if the child were to take 5 mL PO t.i.d.?

$$150 \text{ mL}\left(\frac{1 \text{ dose}}{5 \text{ mL}}\right)\left(\frac{1 \text{ day}}{3 \text{ doses}}\right) = 10 \text{ days}$$

7) A patient has an order for azithromycin 500 mg IV administered over 60 minutes at a concentration of 1 mg/mL. The 500 mg vial states: Prepare the initial solution of azithromycin for injection by adding 4.8 mL of Sterile Water For Injection to the vial and shaking the vial until all of the drug is dissolved. Each mL of the solution contains 100 mg of azithromycin.

a) The 5 mL vial will now be added to what size bag of NS to achieve a 1 mg/mL concentration?

$$500 \text{ mg}\left(\frac{1 \text{ mL}}{\text{mg}}\right) = 500 \text{ mL}$$

b) At what rate will you set the IV infusion pump to the nearest tenth mL/h?

$$\frac{500 \text{ mL}}{60 \text{ min}}\left(\frac{60 \text{ min}}{\text{h}}\right) = \frac{500 \text{ mL}}{\text{h}}$$

8) A patient has an order for streptomycin 500 mg IM which is available in 1 g vials with instructions to add 3.2 mL of Water for Injection USP for a final concentration of 250 mg/mL. How many mL will you administer?

$$500 \text{ mg} \left(\frac{1 \text{ mL}}{250 \text{ mg}}\right) = 2 \text{ mL}$$

9) You have an order for 250 mg IM of a drug which is available in a 500 mg vial with instructions to add 4.3 mL of SW for injection for a final concentration of 100 mg/mL. How many mL will you administer?

$$250 \text{ mg} \left(\frac{1 \text{ mL}}{100 \text{ mg}}\right) = 2.5 \text{ mL}$$

10) The physician has ordered 200 mg IM of a drug which is available in 1 g vials with instructions to add 3.5 mL SW for injection for a final concentration of 250 mg/mL. How many mL will you administer?

$$200 \text{ mg} \left(\frac{1 \text{ mL}}{250 \text{ mg}}\right) = 0.8 \text{ mL}$$

Chapter 23
Conversions Between mg and mEq

1) How many g of sodium acetate are in 16 mEq of sodium acetate?

$$16\ \text{mEq}\left(\frac{1\ \text{mmol}}{\text{mEq}}\right)\left(\frac{82\ \text{mg}}{\text{mmol}}\right)\left(\frac{1\ \text{g}}{1000\ \text{mg}}\right) = 1.31\ \text{g}$$

2) How many grams of Na$^+$ (just the sodium) are contained in 2.5 L of 10% NaCl?

$$2.5\ \text{L}\left(\frac{10\ \text{g NaCl}}{100\ \text{mL}}\right)\left(\frac{1000\ \text{mL}}{\text{L}}\right)\left(\frac{23\ \text{g Na}^+}{58.5\ \text{g NaCl}}\right) = 98.3\ \text{g Na}^+$$

3) How many mEq of NaCl are in 3 L of 0.9% NaCl?

$$3\ \text{L}\left(\frac{0.9\ \text{g}}{100\ \text{mL}}\right)\left(\frac{1000\ \text{mL}}{\text{L}}\right)\left(\frac{1000\ \text{mg}}{\text{g}}\right)\left(\frac{1\ \text{mmol}}{58.5\ \text{mg}}\right)\left(\frac{1\ \text{mEq}}{\text{mmol}}\right) = 461.5\ \text{mEq}$$

4) How many mEq of calcium chloride are contained in 1.5 g of calcium chloride?

$$1.5\ \text{g}\left(\frac{1000\ \text{mg}}{\text{g}}\right)\left(\frac{1\ \text{mmol}}{111.1\ \text{mg}}\right)\left(\frac{2\ \text{mEq}}{\text{mmol}}\right) = 27\ \text{mEq}$$

5) How many mEq of Ca^{++} are in 2.4 g of calcium chloride?

$$2.4\ \text{g}\left(\frac{1000\ \text{mg}}{\text{g}}\right)\left(\frac{1\ \text{mmol}}{111.1\ \text{mg}}\right)\left(\frac{2\ \text{mEq}}{\text{mmol}}\right) = 43.2\ \text{mEq}$$

6) How many mEq of K$^+$ are contained in 240 mg of KCl?

$$240\ \text{mg}\left(\frac{1\ \text{mmol}}{74.6\ \text{mg}}\right)\left(\frac{1\ \text{mEq}}{\text{mmol}}\right) = 3.2\ \text{mEq}$$

7) How many mg of magnesium sulfate are in 20 mEq of magnesium sulfate?

$$20\ \text{mEq}\left(\frac{1\ \text{mmol}}{2\ \text{mEq}}\right)\left(\frac{120.4\ \text{mg}}{\text{mmol}}\right) = 1204\ \text{mg}$$

8) How many mEq of KCl are in 15 mL of 10% KCl solution?

$$15\ \text{mL}\left(\frac{10\ \text{g}}{100\ \text{mL}}\right)\left(\frac{1000\ \text{mg}}{\text{g}}\right)\left(\frac{1\ \text{mmol}}{74.6\ \text{mg}}\right)\left(\frac{1\ \text{mEq}}{\text{mmol}}\right) = 20.1\ \text{mEq}$$

9) How many mEq of MgSO$_4$ are contained in 14 g of MgSO$_4$?

$$14\ \text{g}\left(\frac{1000\ \text{mg}}{\text{g}}\right)\left(\frac{1\ \text{mmol}}{120.4\ \text{mg}}\right)\left(\frac{2\ \text{mEq}}{\text{mmol}}\right) = 232.6\ \text{mEq}$$

10) How many mg of KCl are in 30 mL of 2 mEq/mL KCl?

$$30\ \text{mL}\left(\frac{2\ \text{mEq}}{\text{mL}}\right)\left(\frac{1\ \text{mmol}}{\text{mEq}}\right)\left(\frac{74.6\ \text{mg}}{\text{mmol}}\right) = 4476\ \text{mg}$$

Chapter 24
Dosage Calculations Puzzles

These problems are just for fun and would never happen in a clinical setting. Also, they don't count as part of the 777 questions, so you are still getting your money's worth if you don't do them.

1) You have an order for 1 g of a drug to infuse over 2 hours. The pharmacy sends you a 1 L bag with a note saying: This bag contains 250 mL of 2 mg/mL, 250 mL of 1 mg/mL, 250 mL of 5 mg/mL and 250 mL of NS.

a) At what rate will you set the pump?

Step 1) Calculate the amount of drug in the 1 L bag.

$$250 \text{ mL} \left(\frac{2 \text{ mg}}{\text{mL}}\right) = 500 \text{ mg}$$

$$250 \text{ mL} \left(\frac{1 \text{ mg}}{\text{mL}}\right) = 250 \text{ mg}$$

$$250 \text{ mL} \left(\frac{5 \text{ mg}}{\text{mL}}\right) = 1250 \text{ mg}$$

$$250 \text{ mL} \left(\frac{0 \text{ mg}}{\text{mL}}\right) = 0 \text{ mg}$$

Total is 2000 mg/1000 mL

Step 2) Calculate the volume in mL which contains 1 g.

$$1 \text{ g} \left(\frac{1000 \text{ mg}}{\text{g}}\right)\left(\frac{1000 \text{ mL}}{2000 \text{ mg}}\right) = 500 \text{ mL}$$

You would infuse 500 mL over 2 hours which is 250 mL/h.

b) You started the infusion at 1300. You check on the patient at 1400 only to learn that the patient turned off the pump at 1330 because his friend told him that he didn't need any big pharm drugs. After explaining the importance of the drug to the patient, you get out your calculator and note pad. At what rate will you set the pump to finish the 1 g infusion on time if you restart the infusion at 1345?

At 1330, 125 mL would have been infused, leaving 375 mL. You would have to infuse the 375 mL over 1 hour 15 minutes to finish by 1500.

$$\frac{375 \text{ mL}}{1.25 \text{ h}} = \frac{300 \text{ mL}}{\text{h}}$$

You would set the pump at 300 mL/h and discontinue it at 1500.

2) You have an order to start an IV infusion at x mL/h, where 6x + 40 = 100, on your patient Mr. Smith. The IV bag contains y mg/z mL, where 2y + z = 1500 and z-y = 750. Mr. Smith weighs 83 kg. How many mcg/kg/min is Mr. Smith receiving?

Step 1) Solve for x in the equation 6x + 40 = 100.

6x = 60

X= 10.

You will start the infusion at 10 mL/h.

Step 2) Solve for y and z.

2y + z = 1500

z = 1500 – 2y

Plug 1500 -2y for z in the equation z-y = 750

1500 – 2y – y = 750

-3y = -750

y = 250

z – 250 = 750

z = 1000

The IV bag would contain 250 mg/1000 mL

$$\frac{10\ \text{mL}}{\text{h}}\left(\frac{250\ \text{mg}}{1000\ \text{mL}}\right)\left(\frac{1000\ \text{mcg}}{\text{mg}}\right)\left(\frac{1\ \text{h}}{60\ \text{min}}\right)\left(\frac{1}{83\ \text{kg}}\right) = \frac{0.5\ \text{mcg}}{\text{kg min}}$$

Answer: 0.5 mcg/kg/min

3) A new miracle drug is released by the FDA which reverses aging by 25% in adults over 50 YO. The dosage is 2 mg/kg + 1.5 mg for each year over 50 years old, rounded to the nearest 10 mg, given IV over 2 hours. The drug is available in 10 mg vials with instructions to reconstitute each vial with 8 mL of supplied diluent to yield a concentration of 1 mg/mL. Your facility's protocol is to reconstitute the appropriate number of vials and add to a 500 mL bag of D5W after withdrawing an equal volume of reconstituted drug from the 500 mL bag, then infuse over 2 hours. The drug, Gobakntime, is very expensive at $200/mg. Your facility has a new policy stating that the nurse who administers the drug must also calculate the charge of the drug and collect the cash payment. Your patient, Auld Guy, is 64 years old and weighs 82 kg. He is a little concerned about the price of the drug and relays to you that he makes $23.50/hour as a professional dog food taster. Auld Guy works 8 hours/day, five days per week. What will be the total charge for Auld Guy's therapy and how many weeks, days and hours will he have to work to pay for it?

Step 1) Calculate the total number of mg needed.

82 kg (2 mg/kg) = 164 mg

14 years (1.5 mg/year) = 21 mg

Total = 164 mg + 21 mg = 185 mg rounded to 190 mg

Step 2) Calculate the cost of 190 mg at $200/mg.

190 mg ($200/mg) = $38,000

Step 3) Calculate the number of hours Mr. Guy must work at $23.50/h to make $38,000.

$38,000 (1 h/$23.50) = 1617 h

Step 4) Convert 1617 h to weeks at 40 h/week.

1617 h (1 week/40 h) = 40.425 weeks.

40 weeks = 1600 h, leaving 17 h, which is two 8-hour days plus 1 h.

Answer to total charge for therapy: $38,000.

Answer to how long Mr. Guy must work: 40 weeks, 2 days, 1 h.

Chapter 25
Self-Assessment Exam

Convert the following:

1) 50 mL = **0.05 L**

2) 6.5 g = **6500 mg**

3) 3 tbs = **45 mL**

4) 1 cup = **240 mL**

5) 90 mL = **3 fl oz**

6) 182 lb = **82.7 kg**

7) 6.5 cm = **2.6 in**

8) 0.85 kg = **1.87 lb**

9) 150 g = **0.15 kg**

10) 3 tbs = **45 mL**

Round the following numbers to the nearest tenth.

11) 6.45   **6.5**

12) 0.175   **0.2**

13) 8.97   **9.0**

14) 0.0002   **0.0**

15) 98.045   **98.0**

Round the following numbers to the nearest hundredth.

16) 6.875   **6.88**

17) 4.058   **4.06**

18) 30.005   **30.01**

19) 0.0555   **0.06**

20) 2.178   **2.18**

Write the corresponding Roman numerals for the following numbers:

21) 4   **IV**

22) 9   **IX**

23) 20   **XX**

24) 53   **LIII**

25) 120   **CXX**

Write the corresponding numbers for the following Roman numerals:

26) VII   **7**

27) XIX   **19**

28) XXX   **30**

29) CIX   **109**

30) CCX   **210**

Convert the following to scientific notation:

31) 780,000   **7.8 X 10^5**

32) 142,000,000   **1.42 X 10^8**

33) 0.00054   **5.4 X 10^{-4}**

34) 450   **4.5 X 10^2**

35) 549,000   **5.49 X 10^5**

Convert the following from scientific notation to numbers.

36) 5.34 X 10^4 **53,400**

37) 9.352 X 10^6 **9,352,000**

38) 1.502 X 10^{-5} **0.00001502**

39) 5.1 X 10^{-6} **0.0000051**

40) 2.004 X 10^7 **20,040,000**

Answer the following questions concerning military time.

41) You started studying for your exam at 1900 and finished at 2230. How many hours and minutes did you study?

3 h 30 min

42) What is 3:25 PM in military time?

1525

43) You start and IV at 1000 which is scheduled to run 8 hours. What time will it end in military time?

1800

44) A patient is to receive a medication every 8 hours around the clock. He received doses at 0600 and 1400. When should he receive the next dose?

2200

45) You are asked to work from 11:00 AM to 1800. Your employer tells you that you can either be paid $35.00 per hour or a flat rate of $265. Which is the better deal for you?

Take the $265.   7 h ($35.00/h) = $245.00

Convert the following numbers to percents.

46) 0.05   **0.05 (100%) = 5%**

47) 1.25   **1.25 (100%) = 125%**

48) 0.45   **0.45 (100%) = 45%**

Convert the following percents to numbers.

49) 23.1%   **(23.1%/100%) = 0.231**

50) 100%   **(100%/100%) = 1**

51) 0.15%   **(0.15%/100%) = 0.0015**

Express the following as percent strength solutions and include the type of solution (w/w, w/v, v/v, v/w).

52) 9 g NaCl in 1000 mL   **(9 g/1000 mL)100% = 0.9% w/v**

53) 1 g KCl in 10 mL   **(1 g/10 mL)100% = 10% w/v**

54) 40 mL ETOH in 160 mL. **(40 mL/160 mL)100% = 25% v/v**

Answer the following:

55) How many mg of lidocaine are in 200 mL of 1% lidocaine solution?

200 mL (1 g/100 mL) (1000 mg/g) = 2000 mg

56) How many mg of triamcinolone are in 30 g of 0.5% triamcinolone cream?

30 g (0.5 g Al/100 g) (1000 mg Al/g Al) = 150 mg

57) How many mg of NaCl are in 500 mL of 0.9% NaCl?

500 mL (0.9 g/100 mL) (1000 mg/g) = 4500 mg

Answer the following questions pertaining to percent change.

58) You weigh 160 lb on August 1st and spend the next week hiking around Yosemite National Park. On August 8th you weigh 152 lb. What is the percent change in your weight?

((152-160)/160) 100% = -5%

59) You have two hamsters who fall in love and have 3 babies. What is the percent change in your hamster population?

((5-2)/2) 100% = 150%

60) The physician changed a patient's dose of a drug from 50 mg to 25 mg. What is the percent change in the dose?

((25-50)/50) 100% = -50%

61) Kristina F., a nursing student, scored 80% on her dosage calculation quiz on Monday. The following Monday she scored 90%. What is the percent change in her grade?

((90-80)/80) 100% = 12.5%

62) Your patient weighed 75 kg on admission and now weighs 72 kg. What is the percent change in the patient's weight?

((72-75)/75) 100% = -4%

Answer the following dosage questions.

63) The PCP has ordered 100 mg IM of a drug which is available in 200 mg/mL. How many mL will you administer?

$$100 \text{ mg} \left(\frac{1 \text{ mL}}{200 \text{ mg}} \right) = 0.5 \text{ mL}$$

64) The physician has ordered 30 mg IV of a drug which is available in 5 mL vials of 10 mg/mL. How many mL will you administer?

$$30 \text{ mg} \left(\frac{1 \text{ mL}}{10 \text{ mg}} \right) = 3 \text{ mL}$$

65) The NP ordered 50 mg PO once daily for a patient. The drug is available in 25 mg tablets. How many tablets will the patient take each day?

$$50 \text{ mg} \left(\frac{1 \text{ tab}}{25 \text{ mg}} \right) = 2 \text{ tabs}$$

66) The physician has ordered 90 mg IM of a drug which is available in 5 mL vials containing 45 mg/mL. How many mL will you administer?

$$90 \text{ mg} \left(\frac{1 \text{ mL}}{45 \text{ mg}} \right) = 2 \text{ mL}$$

67) Your patient has an order for 12.5 mg PO of a drug which is available in 5 mg scored tablets. How many tabs will you administer?

$$12.5 \text{ mg} \left(\frac{1 \text{ tab}}{5 \text{ mg}} \right) = 2.5 \text{ tabs}$$

68) Your 52 YO patient, who weighs 165 lb, has an order for drug xyz 100 mg/day divided into two doses. Drug xyz is available in 10 mL vials containing 50 mg/mL. How many mL will you administer per dose?

$$\frac{100 \text{ mg}}{\text{day}} \left(\frac{1 \text{ day}}{2 \text{ doses}} \right) \left(\frac{1 \text{ mL}}{50 \text{ mg}} \right) = \frac{1 \text{ mL}}{\text{dose}}$$

69) You have an order to administer 100 mcg/day PO divided into two doses. You have 0.025 mg tablets available. How many tablets will you administer per dose?

$$\frac{100 \text{ mcg}}{\text{day}} \left(\frac{1 \text{ day}}{2 \text{ doses}} \right) \left(\frac{1 \text{ tab}}{0.025 \text{ mg}} \right) \left(\frac{1 \text{ mg}}{1000 \text{ mcg}} \right) = \frac{2 \text{ tabs}}{\text{dose}}$$

70) Your patient has an order for 250 mg IV every 6 hours of a drug which is available in 10 mL vials containing 25 mg/mL. How many mL will be administered in 24 hours?

$$\frac{1000 \text{ mg}}{24 \text{ h}} \left(\frac{1 \text{ mL}}{25 \text{ mg}} \right) = \frac{40 \text{ mL}}{24 \text{ h}}$$

71) The physician has ordered 250 mcg IM of a drug which is available in 2 mL vials containing 0.5 mg/mL. How many mL will you administer?

$$250 \text{ mcg} \left(\frac{1 \text{ mL}}{25 \text{ mg}} \right) \left(\frac{1 \text{ mg}}{1000 \text{ mcg}} \right) = 0.5 \text{ mL}$$

72) The physician has ordered 40 mg IV of a drug which is available in 5 mL vials containing 20 mg/mL. How many mL will you administer?

$$40 \text{ mg} \left(\frac{1 \text{ mL}}{20 \text{ mg}} \right) = 2 \text{ mL}$$

73) A 45 lb child has an order for furosemide 2 mg/kg PO once daily. Furosemide oral solution is available in 60 mL bottles containing 10 mg/mL. How many mL will you administer per dose?

$$\left(\frac{2 \text{ mg}}{\text{kg}}\right)\left(\frac{45 \text{ lb}}{1}\right)\left(\frac{1 \text{ kg}}{2.2 \text{ lb}}\right)\left(\frac{1 \text{ mL}}{10 \text{ mg}}\right) = 4.1 \text{ mL}$$

74) An 81 kg patient is to receive an initial bolus dose of a drug 0.085 mg/kg over at least 2 minutes. The drug is available in 4 mL vials containing 2.5 mg/mL. How many mL will you administer?

$$\left(\frac{0.085 \text{ mg}}{\text{kg}}\right)\left(\frac{81 \text{ kg}}{1}\right)\left(\frac{1 \text{ mL}}{2.5 \text{ mg}}\right) = 2.8 \text{ mL}$$

75) A 135 lb patient is to receive a single IV dose of ondansetron 0.15 mg/kg for prevention of nausea and vomiting. Ondansetron is available in 20 mL MDV of 2 mg/mL. How many mL will you administer?

$$\left(\frac{0.15 \text{ mg}}{\text{kg}}\right)\left(\frac{135 \text{ lb}}{1}\right)\left(\frac{1 \text{ kg}}{2.2 \text{ lb}}\right)\left(\frac{1 \text{ mL}}{2 \text{ mg}}\right) = 4.6 \text{ mL}$$

Calculate the flow rate in mL per hour rounded to the nearest tenth mL/h.

76) 1000 mL infused over 8 hours.

$$\frac{1000 \text{ mL}}{8 \text{ h}} = \frac{125 \text{ mL}}{\text{h}}$$

77) 500 mL infused over 7 hours.

$$\frac{500 \text{ mL}}{7 \text{ h}} = \frac{71.4 \text{ mL}}{\text{h}}$$

78) 1000 mL infused over 6 hours.

$$\frac{1000 \text{ mL}}{6 \text{ h}} = \frac{166.7 \text{ mL}}{\text{h}}$$

79) 100 mL infused over 30 minutes.

$$\frac{100 \text{ mL}}{30 \text{ min}}\left(\frac{60 \text{ min}}{\text{h}}\right) = \frac{200 \text{ mL}}{\text{h}}$$

Calculate the flow rate in drops/min. Round to the nearest whole drop.

80) 500 mL infused over 4 hours with a drop factor of 20 (20 gtts/mL).

$$\frac{500 \text{ mL}}{4 \text{ h}}\left(\frac{1 \text{ h}}{60 \text{ min}}\right)\left(\frac{20 \text{ gtts}}{\text{mL}}\right) = \frac{42 \text{ gtts}}{\text{min}}$$

81) 1000 mL infused over 8 hours with a drop factor of 10.

$$\frac{1000 \text{ mL}}{8 \text{ h}}\left(\frac{1 \text{ h}}{60 \text{ min}}\right)\left(\frac{10 \text{ gtts}}{\text{mL}}\right) = \frac{21 \text{ gtts}}{\text{min}}$$

82) 250 mL infused over 2 hours with a drop factor of 15.

$$\frac{250 \text{ mL}}{2 \text{ h}}\left(\frac{1 \text{ h}}{60 \text{ min}}\right)\left(\frac{15 \text{ gtts}}{\text{mL}}\right) = \frac{31 \text{ gtts}}{\text{min}}$$

83) 100 mL infused over 2 hours with a microdrip set (60 gtts/mL).

$$\frac{100 \text{ mL}}{2 \text{ h}}\left(\frac{1 \text{ h}}{60 \text{ min}}\right)\left(\frac{60 \text{ gtts}}{\text{mL}}\right) = \frac{50 \text{ gtts}}{\text{min}}$$

Calculate the length of time in hours and minutes, rounded to the nearest minute, required to infuse the following:

84) 500 mL at 40 mL/h.

$$500 \text{ mL} \left(\frac{1 \text{ h}}{40 \text{ mL}}\right) = 12.5 \text{ h} = 12 \text{ h } 30 \text{ min}$$

85) 1000 mL at 110 mL/h.

$$1000 \text{ mL} \left(\frac{1 \text{ h}}{110 \text{ mL}}\right) = 9.09 \text{ h} = 9 \text{ h } 5 \text{ min}$$

86) 500 mL at 35 gtts/min with a drop factor of 20.

$$500 \text{ mL} \left(\frac{1 \text{ min}}{35 \text{ gtts}}\right)\left(\frac{20 \text{ gtts}}{\text{mL}}\right) = 286 \text{ min} = 4 \text{ h } 46 \text{ min}$$

87) 1 L at 30 gtts/min with a drop factor of 15.

$$1 \text{ L} \left(\frac{1000 \text{ mL}}{\text{L}}\right)\left(\frac{1 \text{ min}}{30 \text{ gtts}}\right)\left(\frac{15 \text{ gtts}}{\text{mL}}\right) = 500 \text{ min} = 8 \text{ h } 20 \text{ min}$$

Calculate the volume infused in the following scenarios.

88) Infusion rate of 30 mL/h for 4 h 30 min.

$$4.5 \text{ h} \left(\frac{30 \text{ mL}}{\text{h}}\right) = 135 \text{ mL}$$

89) Infusion rate of 28 gtts/min, drop factor 20, for 3 hours 15 min.

$$3.25 \text{ h} \left(\frac{28 \text{ gtts}}{\text{min}}\right)\left(\frac{60 \text{ min}}{\text{h}}\right)\left(\frac{1 \text{ mL}}{20 \text{ gtts}}\right) = 273 \text{ mL}$$

Calculate the following. Round all drops/min to the nearest drop and all mL/h rates to the nearest tenth mL/h.

90) Your 67 kg patient has an order for a lidocaine infusion at the rate of 30 mcg/kg/min. You have a 250 mL bag labeled "Lidocaine HCl and 5% Dextrose Injection USP". Lidocaine 2 g (8 mg/mL) is printed in big red letters in the middle of the label. What rate will you set the IV infusion pump?

$$\frac{30 \text{ mcg}}{\text{kg min}}\left(\frac{67 \text{ kg}}{1}\right)\left(\frac{1 \text{ mL}}{8 \text{ mg}}\right)\left(\frac{1 \text{ mg}}{1000 \text{ mcg}}\right)\left(\frac{60 \text{ min}}{\text{h}}\right) = \frac{15.1 \text{ mL}}{\text{h}}$$

91) Your 140 lb patient, who has been diagnosed with septic shock, has an order for norepinephrine 0.15 mcg/kg/min IV. The pharmacy delivers a bag containing 4 mg norepinephrine in 250 mL D5NS. At what rate will you set the IV infusion pump?

$$\frac{0.15 \text{ mcg}}{\text{kg min}}\left(\frac{140 \text{ lb}}{1}\right)\left(\frac{1 \text{ kg}}{2.2 \text{ lb}}\right)\left(\frac{250 \text{ mL}}{4 \text{ mg}}\right)\left(\frac{1 \text{ mg}}{1000 \text{ mcg}}\right)\left(\frac{60 \text{ min}}{\text{h}}\right) = \frac{35.8 \text{ mL}}{\text{h}}$$

92) Your 140 lb female patient has an order for dobutamine 5 mcg/kg/min IV to start at 1100. The dobutamine is available as 1000 mcg/mL. At what rate will you set the IV infusion pump?

$$\frac{5 \text{ mcg}}{\text{kg min}}\left(\frac{140 \text{ lb}}{1}\right)\left(\frac{1 \text{ kg}}{2.2 \text{ lb}}\right)\left(\frac{1 \text{ mL}}{1000 \text{ mcg}}\right)\left(\frac{60 \text{ min}}{\text{h}}\right) = \frac{19.1 \text{ mL}}{\text{h}}$$

Answer the following reconstitution calculation questions.

93) You have an order for 300 mg IM of a drug which is available in 1 g vials with directions to reconstitute with 7.5 mL of SW for injection for a final concentration of 100 mg/mL. How many mL will you administer?

$$300 \text{ mg} \left(\frac{1 \text{ mL}}{100 \text{ mg}}\right) = 3 \text{ mL}$$

94) A patient has an order for 500 mg IM of a drug which is available in 1 g vials with instructions to add 3.1 mL of Water for Injection USP for a final concentration of 250 mg/mL. How many mL will you administer?

$$500 \text{ mg} \left(\frac{1 \text{ mL}}{250 \text{ mg}}\right) = 2 \text{ mL}$$

Calculate the BSA in m² for the following people using the Mosteller formula.

95) An adult male weighing 185 lb and 5 ft 10 in tall.

$$BSA = \sqrt{\frac{185 \times 70}{3131}} = 2.03 \text{ m}^2$$

96) A 14-month-old girl weighing 23 lb and 31 in tall.

$$BSA = \sqrt{\frac{23 \times 31}{3131}} = 0.48 \text{ m}^2$$

97) An adult male weighing 214 lb and 6 ft 2 in tall.

$$BSA = \sqrt{\frac{214 \times 74}{3131}} = 2.25 \text{ m}^2$$

Answer the following:

98) A mEq of Na^+ and a mEq of K^+ weigh the same. T or **F**

False. Since Na^+ and K^+ both have one charge, they will each have the same number of ions per mEq but will have different weights.

99) A mEq of Na^+ and a mEq of K^+ contain the same number of ions. **T** or F

True. Since Na^+ and K^+ both have one charge, they will each have the same number of ions per mEq.

100) Congratulations on finishing the self-assessment exam. It is important to be confident in your dosage calculations. T or F.

True!

Printed in Great Britain
by Amazon